MOVE MORE AT YOUR DESK

Increase Your Energy at
Work & Reduce Back,
Shoulder & Neck Pain

Kerrie-Anne Bradley

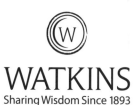

WATKINS
Sharing Wisdom Since 1893

Move More At Your Desk
Kerrie-Anne Bradley

First published in the UK and USA in 2022 by
Watkins, an imprint of Watkins Media Limited
Unit 11, Shepperton House,
83–93 Shepperton Road
London N1 3DF

enquiries@watkinspublishing.com

Commissioning Editor: Anya Hayes
Editorial Assistant: Brittany Willis
Head of Design: Karen Smith
Designer: Kate Cromwell
Illustrator: Johanna Arajuuri
Production: Uzma Taj

A CIP record for this book is available from
the British Library

ISBN: 978-1-786786-07-4 (Paperback)

ISBN: 978-1-786786-23-4 (eBook)

10 9 8 7 6 5 4 3 2 1

Printed in Bosnia and Herzegovina

Disclaimer: All of the movements in
this book are functional and safe. That
said, should anything cause pain you
should stop immediately and consult
your medical practitioner. If you have any
health conditions that are affected by
movement, please consult your medical
professional to identify which movements
are contraindicated, if any.

www.watkinspublishing.com

The movements I share in this book
are movements I have learnt along my
movement journey. I did not invent them.
However, the way that I teach them is in
my own way and words. Where an
exercise is particular to a person I have
had experience working with, I have said.

Contents

Introduction: Let's Get Moving   4

1 What is Movement?   12

2 Sitting and Standing   40

3 The Move More Moves   64

4 Other Ways to Move While You Work   156

5 Setting Yourself Up for More Movement   174

6 Some Suggested Mini Movement Routines   188

Et Voilà!   198
About the Author   199
Acknowledgements   200
Notes   201
Bibliography   203
Useful Resources   206
Index   210

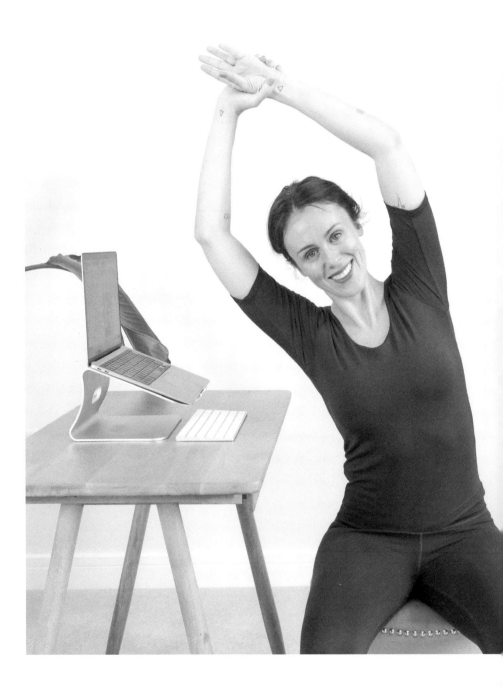

Let's Get Moving

"Movement should be approached like life – with enthusiasm, joy and gratitude – for movement is life, and life is movement, and we get out of it what we put into it."

Ron Fletcher

This is a book about simple ways to move more while you work. It isn't about running around the block 10 times, doing 100 press-ups every hour or jumping in the air and landing in the box splits – it's about small, simple and varied ways to move more so that your body is less stiff, stronger, more energized and feels good.

If you are someone who spends a lot of time sitting at work and/ or a lot of time sitting when not working, then this book is for you. It provides a toolkit of movements for you to try and a practical guide on how to integrate more movement into your day.

The underlying message of this book is that moving around is better for our bodies than staying still for long periods of time. For many of us, though, sitting is a major part of how we work, and so much of our lives is also geared toward sitting these days: eating, commuting, watching TV, scrolling on our phones ... the list could go on!

So, unless we intend to ditch all our chairs and sign up to a seat-free life, we need to think about how we sit. This book will therefore also show you how to sit (and stand!) in an active and balanced way.

Our bodies are designed to move, and can do this in many different ways, and at varying speeds. There is no disputing that for those of us who hold our bodies in a relatively fixed position for several hours a day, introducing a variety of movements is a good thing. The examples in this book will hopefully show you how to explore your movement potential without even having to leave your workspace.

This book is about breaking down the barriers that prevent us from moving, which is why the movements are simple, accessible and quick, and why no special equipment or clothing is needed for them.

The aim is to leave you feeling more informed about moving your body during the day so that you can feel energized, stretched, better aligned, stronger, calmer and hopefully happier. For those of you with desk-related pain, I hope that the advice and suggestions here will leave your body feeling less achy too.

This is a practical guide to moving more at your desk, so I will be asking you to sit on your sit bones (you're going to hear quite a lot about this ...) and FIDGET.

My Movement Journey

My name is Kerrie-Anne, and I am an ex-professional sloucher turned Pilates teacher. I have a business called Pilates At Your Desk (PAYD), where I teach individuals and businesses across the world how to move more and how to sit/stand in a balanced and active way while at work.

Many years working as an economist, sitting like a cross between a pretzel and a croissant (for the non-imagery learners among you, this will be explored later) really took its toll on my body: I had constant shoulder pain, sciatica, an awful lower back and dodgy knees!

I quit my job as an economist and retrained with Fletcher Pilates, which is a Pilates school started by one of the first-generation teachers (meaning that he trained directly with Joseph Pilates himself, who created the method), Ron Fletcher.

So what is Pilates? In short, it is a programme of strength, flexibility and mobility movements looking to bring about better alignment and balance throughout the mind and body. This repertoire of movement

– either performed on a mat or on specially-developed Pilates equipment – was first developed by Joseph Pilates in the early 20th century. In daily life, and indeed in sport, we will use particular parts of our bodies on a repetitive basis. Some parts become overused, while others are underused. Pilates is about getting the parts that do not move as much, moving. It is about working those smaller, deeper muscles and engaging the mind to focus on how to do that.

At the time, I saw the teaching course as a stop gap while I figured out what I would do next, but when I started teaching, I realized I had found my calling. I had been looking at bodies my whole life (lots of time spent on benches eating lunch, watching the world go by). As a result, I had connected lots of dots and could generally figure out why a person was experiencing discomfort or pain, based on how they walked, sat, lay and stood still. So now, instead of working as an economist, I go around applying my problem-solving skills to pelvises and spines. I specialize in alignment and also work with lots of people with limited mobility due to injury or particular medical conditions.

I would describe my approach as somewhat intuitive insofar as I am guided by the body in front of me. I continue my education with regular workshops but, that said, much of the development of my knowledge tends to come from what I learn from those I teach. I base my Pilates lessons on what the body needs. More often than not, when the body is in a place of pain or discomfort, what is required are simple moves and tips on how to change how the body moves, or indeed how it is static, on a daily basis. This is where I see the biggest results in terms of benefits to wellbeing.

In fact, Pilates At Your Desk came about because I was noticing that my desk-based clients would come with new aches and pains week in, week out, even though they would leave me feeling great. So, I put together a very small programme of movements for them to do between lessons: not mat-based, but movements they could do at their desks. Those who did the moves told me how much they benefitted from them; their weekly aches and pains disappeared (or, at least, were significantly muted). This inspired me to develop a business focusing primarily on these small but highly beneficial movement-based changes.

Better body awareness, being more aligned, breathing more efficiently and (of course) incorporating more movement has made a massive difference to me and to the many bodies I work with through one-to-ones, group and corporate teaching.

I have worked with tech giants, law firms, accountancy firms, banks, advertising agencies, PR companies, media companies, fashion brands, NHS nurses, NHS radiologists and radiographers, hairdressing salons and even breweries. The result is always the same: more movement, and moving well, makes people feel better.

Movement in a Pandemic

At the time of writing this book, the world was in the midst of the COVID-19 crisis and lockdown. Working from home was the new norm and, as a result, the majority of those who worked at desks were moving less. The commute to work had become a thing of the past. As had walking across the office or popping out for a coffee. We had become a nation of office-at-home workers experiencing back-to-back meetings, with little time or space to move.

The number of online Pilates At Your Desk workshops I was being booked to teach increased dramatically. Businesses were recognizing that staff were moving less, sitting at their desks for longer periods of time and more people were reporting aches and pains.

Also, many of the businesses I was working with did not know what the "new normal" would look like on the other side of the pandemic. I heard many reports of businesses asking people to mix up working at home and at the office to a greater extent. Some businesses would return to full time in the office, while others would now have their staff permanently work from home.

Given this uncertainty, I have included information on both scenarios: working from home and working in the office. The movements are the same in both cases (although some may be a bit "out there" for the office ... unless everyone is doing it and it's culturally acceptable to be a big star and a little ball – see page 101!). The differences lie more in the tips I give on when to integrate more movement. Whatever your situation, I'm sure you'll find them useful.

Not Just for Those With Desk Jobs

Despite the name, I want to emphasize that the movements in this book are great for everyone, and not just those with desk jobs. I've worked with many groups of people who predominantly stand to work, including, for example, NHS nurses, pharmacists and brewery workers, and I have included experiences from some of these people in the book, along with those from other sectors who mainly find themselves sitting at work.

The moves I outline can work for anyone who finds themselves in certain positions for long periods at a time and/or doing repetitive movements with the same body parts over and over each day. I'll also show you how it is possible to stand in an active and balanced way.

A Movement for Workplace Movement

My mission is to get as many people as I can moving more during the day. This is why I teach corporate workshops and offer daily movement videos on Instagram (@pilatesatyourdesk). However, a workplace where everyone is encouraged to move more is what I am ultimately aiming for. Yes, it is about individuals being accountable for how much they move (with help from me!), but the bigger picture is making this movement something that is culturally embedded into the workplace, so that it becomes a place where you are actively encouraged to move. Workplace productivity goes up when people move more and feel better in their bodies, and increased productivity is good for business – it's a win-win situation.

So let's make this movement a workplace movement.

Actually, stuff it – let's go global!

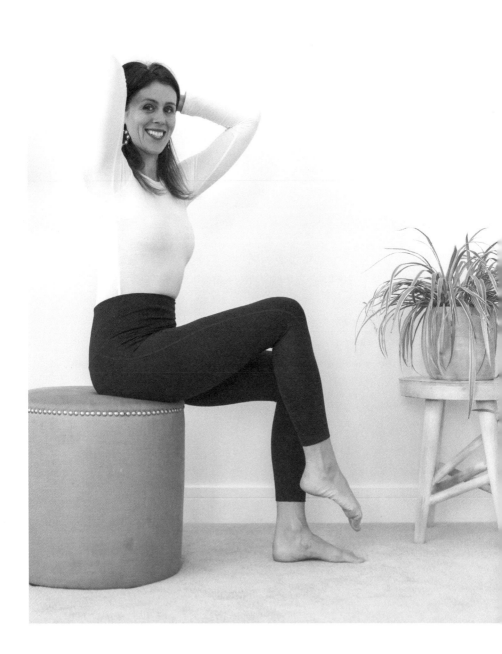

chapter 1.

What is Movement?

Movement is motion: every time you change the position of any body part, you are moving. It is what we do to get things done. It is also what we do to feel good (this may not be the first thing that springs to your mind, but hopefully, after reading this book, that will change).

Wiggling your little finger is movement. Stretching your arms above your head is movement. Looking over your shoulder is movement. Standing up and down is movement. Squatting is movement. Blinking is movement. Running 10k is movement.

For the more scientific of you, movement – or physical activity (which I will use interchangeably here) – can be defined as "any bodily movement produced by skeletal muscles that results in energy expenditure".[1] Basically, if we have to use energy to do it, it counts as movement.

Humans have the potential to move in many different ways, at different speeds and for different amounts of time. We are hugely capable creatures in this respect! In fact, there are so many different ways in which you can move your body that I am not even sure it would be possible to count the number of permutations. (At the time of writing this, even Google couldn't come up with an answer to this question.)

What Movement is Covered in This Book

This book looks at ways of moving your body while you are at work, so it predominantly covers seated and standing movements you can do at your desk.

Opposite are some of the ways we will move in this book.

Move More at Your Desk focuses on moving your body in gentle ways through stretching, mobilizing and strengthening all of your body parts, and is about helping your body work in a more balanced way, recognizing that we often tend to hold particular positions as we work. The movements in this book get the body

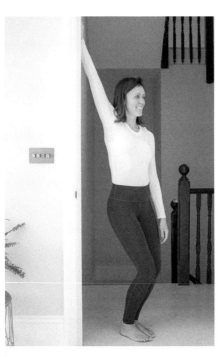
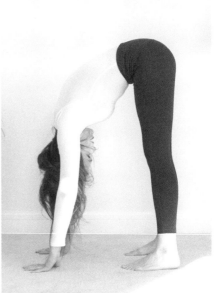
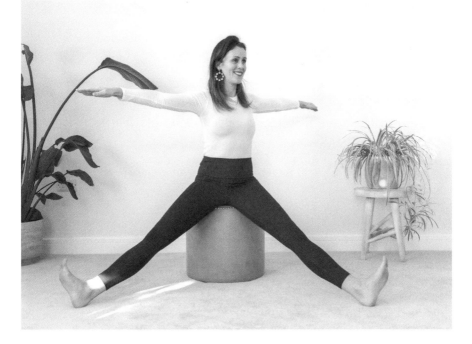

working in different ways that can help counter these tendencies and help us to utilize our muscles more evenly.

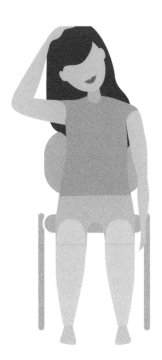

You could describe this type of movement as incidental, and indeed a key aim of this book is to provide ways that can help increase the extent to which we engage in healthy movement more incidentally while working. In line with this, I will provide you with small amounts of varied movement that can be done on a regular basis throughout the day, and that can be incorporated into your work (and home life) routines. Some practical ideas for how to do this are provided in Chapter 5, and you will also discover some of the inventive ways my clients have come up with for integrating movement into their working days in the various case studies I have included throughout the book.

Movement and exercise

One type of movement you may do – when not at work, I would assume – is longer bursts of planned, repetitive, structured movement. This is more commonly known as "exercise".

Emma Bray (see page 208), a fellow movement expert, shared these thoughts about the term "exercise", and I have to agree with her:

> *"We have labelled movement as exercise, with exercise being a set time repeating movements, but the reality is we 'exercise' all the time. It's semantics, a mindset, and perhaps not a helpful one for most of us."*

Indeed, the word "movement" has over time tended to become synonymous with the word "exercise" when, in fact, planned and structured exercise is just one way of moving.

With so many of us being time-poor, this focus on "exercise" can mean that, in practice, we end up moving less than we would if we approached it differently and thought, for example, *Ah – I have two minutes before my next meeting. I'll wiggle my body a bit while I wait.*

Perhaps a key first step in this quest for more movement is changing how we talk about it. Instead of thinking of movement as being something for which you need to carve out time, change clothes, go somewhere special or follow a routine to do, perhaps we should think more of it as something you can do *at any time* and *in any place.*

YOUR BODY!

I thought it might be helpful at this point, for the more scientifically minded of you, to set out an overview of the key body terms involved in movement. Following this I provide a summary of what happens when you move.

SKELETON – This is the structure of bones and joint systems within the body that houses your organs.

BONES – An adult has 206 bones, and they are different shapes and sizes, depending on their function – the biggest being your upper leg bone (femur) and the smallest being a wee one in your ear. The bones protect your organs, store calcium and fat and produce blood cells. Most importantly in relation to this book, our bones provide attachment sites for muscles and so create a structure that supports movement.

JOINTS – This is where bones articulate with each other. Joints come in different shapes and sizes, enabling different types of movement. Some allow a greater range of movement, (e.g. the ball and socket joints in your shoulders and hips) whereas others can only move on a single plane (e.g. the hinge joints of your knees).

MUSCLES – There are over 600 muscles in your body, and they all come in different shapes and sizes. These are the guys that contract and relax, enabling you to move, sit up and stay still. There are also different kinds of muscle – in this book, we are referring to our skeletal muscles, which, as the name suggests, are attached to our skeleton.

FASCIA – Fascia refers to the connective tissue that is woven throughout the entire body. It can be thin and delicate surrounding organs, muscles or blood vessels, or thick and tough like the Plantar Fascia on the sole of your foot.

NERVOUS SYSTEM – Your nervous system is like your body's central control hub that controls everything you do. It comprises your brain, spinal cord and all of the nerves in your body.

How Do We Move?

Here is a short trip down anatomy lane to (re)familiarize yourself with what happens in the body whenever we make a movement.

We have control over some types of movement and not others. There are certain bodily functions that are autonomous – for example, your heart beating – that thankfully we don't have to remember to do. However, the types of movement we are looking at in this book are ones that are *voluntary*. That is, where there needs to be some sort of stimulus that creates a response from the brain in order to action a movement. Here is a very high-level summary of how this works.

- When you action a movement, a signal from your brain is sent to the muscles needed via the nervous system telling the muscle(s) that it/they are needed for action.

- The muscle fibres contract, moving the bone(s) in question.

- To relax the muscles, another signal is sent.

- The bones in question return to their resting position.

To delve a bit deeper into this, it is relevant to next turn our minds to the wonderful world of fascia. We used to look at the body as a system of individual parts, but more recently, anatomical research has identified that our bodies are more complex than this. In fact, there is a system of connective tissue integrating the whole body, connecting everything, called fascia.

FASCIA

Movement teacher and educator Kath Pentecost (see page 208) knows more about fascia than I do and is a great source of information. I quizzed her on what happens connective-tissue-wise when we move, and she told me this:

"Fascia refers to the body-wide, tensional network of connective tissue in the human body that is form-giving, force-transmitting and sensory-rich. It quite literally connects everything to everything and – fun fact – your fascial system would show the shape of your body when viewed independently (if this was possible), much like your circulatory system and nervous system.

The term fascia includes a number of different types of connective tissue. Your tendons and ligaments are all parts of your fascial network, as well as fascia that wraps around your muscles and, to go one step further, even your muscle fibres are embedded in fascia. Every single movement we make involves both muscles and fascia, so they cannot be separated. Instead, we can train both deliberately by changing the focus of what we do.

This is very significant in terms of movement. Firstly, to look at the body's anatomy in a more integrated way makes a lot of sense. Bear in mind we can never truly isolate one muscle or one joint without influencing this body-wide network. Just like when a fly lands on a spider's web, it is the whole web that moves, or how your whole T-shirt moves when you pull on the corner of it, when you move one part of your body, the whole body responds fascially to that movement. Its unique architecture also means that our tensional, web-like network of fascia is strong, elastic and adaptable, with different specializations in different areas of the body as required. Remember, form follows function, and our fascia adapts in response to the way we use our bodies.

Fascia consist of fibres, ground substance (gel-like and absorbent material), water and cells. Therefore, hydration is one key quality of fascia. When it comes to movement, we can compare fascia to a sponge that is being rehydrated when we move. As areas of tissue become stretched or tensioned, this fluid is squeezed out; on release, as the tissue softens again, it becomes rehydrated and refreshed. Such a simple concept, but the effects are far-reaching.

So, keep moving and remember your fascial system loves multi-directional movement of varying intensities to maintain its inherent resilience and adaptability."

How Much Should We Be Moving?

"Lack of activity destroys the good condition of every human being, while movement and methodical physical exercise save it and preserve it."

Plato

In short, the answer to how much we should be moving is: **as much and in as many different ways as possible.**

In terms of regular movement, it is widely accepted that for every 20–30 minutes you sit, you should move for a few minutes. This is what I tend to recommend to people. That said, any movement is better than none, and if every 20–30 minutes does not work for you, then find out what does.

And remember – it all counts. We need to forget this idea of movement only counting if we set aside an hour to do it. Even that little wiggle on your chair – that you might do now as you read this! – is still an excellent movement choice for you to make.

In fact, in 2020, the World Health Organization published an article entitled "Every move counts toward better health", and suggested that adults should be doing 150–300 minutes of *moderate to vigorous* movement per week, which adds up to less than an hour per day. "All physical activity is beneficial," the report said, "and can be done as part of work, sport and leisure or transport (walking ... and cycling), but also through dance, play and everyday household tasks, like gardening and cleaning."[2] Arguably they could have added in "while working at your desk", but hey, perhaps they will do next time around! For now, the fact that this statement includes so much more than just busting it out in the gym is a good start.

A WORD FROM
PROFESSOR FEHMIDAH MUNIR

Professor Fehmidah Munir (see page 209) is a professor of Health Psychology at Loughborough University. Her current research focuses on the promotion of health and management of wellbeing in occupational settings. This work includes research into sedentary behaviour – most notably the 36-month research project, "Stand More AT (SMArT) Work".

I came across Professor Munir when putting together material for my corporate workshops. I asked her to comment on her research around the impacts of being sedentary and how often we should be moving. You will find comments from Fehmidah throughout the book. In terms of how often we should be moving, here is some evidence supporting the view that we should be breaking up sitting with movement every 30 minutes:

"Research has found that frequently breaking up excessive sitting with physical activity has huge positive effects.[3] Experimental studies show that breaking up prolonged sitting with short but frequent bouts of light-intensity physical activity (e.g. standing, walking, stretches, squats) over a 6–8-hour time period reduces blood glucose levels, insulin, body fat and blood pressure compared to prolonged sitting with no breaks.[456] In terms of time, this means taking breaks every 20–30 minutes for up to five minutes at a time throughout the working day.

A consensus statement by physical activity experts[7] recommends that workers should initially aim toward 'accumulating two hours a day of standing and light activity (light walking) during working hours, eventually progressing to a total accumulation of four hours per day (prorated to part-time hours)'. As sitting is often accrued in prolonged periods of over 30 minutes,[8] this means breaking up sitting time by standing and doing some light movement every half hour or so."

The upshot is: the more you do, the better it is for you. Weaving it into your everyday life so that it becomes part of what you do is key here, and if you can move at your desk while you work, then this is a good thing. Some physical activity is better than doing none, but by becoming more active throughout the day in relatively simple ways, people can easily achieve the recommended activity levels.

DON'T SET YOURSELF UP FOR FAILURE

There is a common trend in the fitness world that classes last one hour. However, as far as I can tell, this length of time has come about more because it makes it easier for the industry – and us – to timetable and structure our days than because it's the optimal amount of time to exercise.

I was speaking to a client about this last week who said that she knows that she does not have time to always do an hour, but psychologically feels she should. So, rather setting herself up for failure, she doesn't do any movement at all.

If you feel this way too, you shouldn't. The WHO guidelines, at the lower end, mean that even 30 minutes of movement a day is fab, and you can accrue that in short bursts. Obviously more is better, but it all adds up.

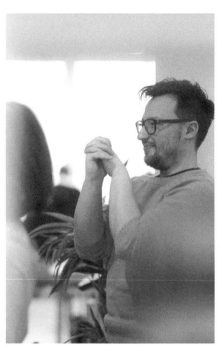
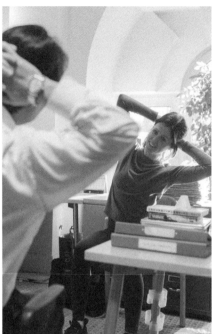
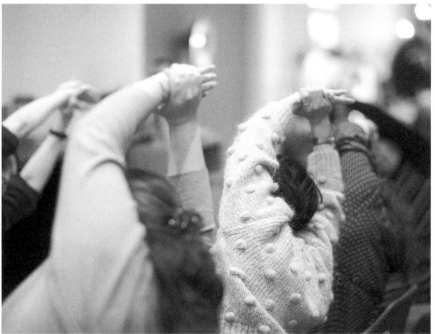

The Movement Bank

In my corporate workshops I like to talk about us each having our own movement bank. It's a very simplistic analogy that doesn't account for any variability in credit between different types of movement, but it serves well as an illustration.

For each one of us:

- Movement is a **credit**

- Being sedentary (having long, uninterrupted periods of sitting) is a **debit**

So, the more movement you do, the more credit you get in the bank. The more sitting you do, the more debits are taken from the bank The likelihood is that different sorts of movement will hold different amounts of credit, and this would also be true of different lengths of time that you are moving for. But what is also true is that the higher the number of times you move throughout the day, the lower the debits you'll have, and so the more likely you are to be in credit by the end of the working day.

So, even though a longer workout may give you more credit than, say, a number of short movement breaks, if you are sitting for the majority of the rest of the time when you are awake, then that credit may not be enough to offset the debits you have accrued, and you may still be in a movement deficit. Given this, the more incidental movement you do – including by making more movement more incidental – the better. Of course, we will be more motivated to do this under some circumstances rather than others, e.g. where the movement enables us to do something else. But I'm hoping that by the end of this book you'll be motivated to try to integrate more movement into your work and home-life routines, to help your movement bank to always be in credit.

Remember, whether it's wiggling your fingers, turning your head from side to side or marching your legs while you sit – it all counts.

Assuming we all prefer leisure over work time, accruing movement credit during the working day can mean that by the time you finish work, you've got heaps of credit in the bank. Consequently, there's less need to go beat yourself up before bed, or to feel guilty about catching up on Netflix (although I would also encourage you to take small movement breaks during this too – but more on that later on in the book). So why is it so good to get credit in the movement bank?

Movement is Good For You

Movement is good for you for so many reasons. Here are some reasons to move:

Movement is Good For Your Muscles and Bones

First up, moving your body strengthens your muscles and makes them more flexible. We need our muscles to be strong and flexible to help us move well and be pain-free. Moving also mobilizes your joints. Movement also helps with balance, which is particularly useful as it helps prevent us from falling.

We need our bones to be strong too, which movement, in particular weight-bearing and muscle-strengthening movement – even the low-intensity kind – does. Our bones are living tissues and the more we use them, the stronger they get.

Subtle movement throughout the day can help your body feel less stiff by hydrating your connective tissue, so that when you do engage in more intense activity, you are less likely to hurt yourself because your body parts are able to move around more fluidly.

Movement is Good For Your Energy

Movement is a natural energy booster. The more you move, the more energy you will have, so eventually you'll feel ready for a little more. There is a positive correlation between physical activity and energy, and also a negative one in that the converse is also true: the more sedentary you are, the less energy you have.

Movement is Good For Your Health

According to the World Health Organization in their 2020 study into physical activity and being sedentary, all levels of physical activity, including light activity, are associated with a lower risk of death. More movement reduces the risk of many health issues, including cardiovascular issues, type-2 diabetes and certain types of cancer.[9]

Movement is Good For Your Mind

It is widely accepted that movement is good for the mind and that the more you move, the happier you feel! Even small amounts of movement can have a positive effect on how you feel. In fact,

A WORD FROM
PROFESSOR FEHMIDAH MUNIR

"Research carried out by myself and others from Loughborough University and the University of Leicester showed that reducing sitting time by as little as one hour every day can benefit many aspects of health and be cost-saving for employers.

Our research study, called Stand More AT (SMArT) Work, found that when office workers were provided with a programme of education and resources encouraging less sitting throughout the workday (motivational posters, apps and software to enable their employees to track sitting time and get reminders to stand up more regularly, advice on how to make small environmental changes), they sat 82 minutes less per day compared to those who did not receive the programme.

Positive changes to the health of those who sat less were observed, including reduced feelings of fatigue and musculoskeletal issues, such as lower back pain, reduced levels of sickness presenteeism at work and improvements in quality of life, work performance, work dedication and engagement."

research studies looking at mental health and sitting time have shown that breaking up excessive sitting time with light activity may reduce depression symptoms by 10 per cent and anxiety by 15 per cent.[10]

I recently listened to an episode of Dr Rangan Chatterjee's podcast, "Feel Better Live More: How 10 minutes of exercise a day can improve your mental health",[11] in which Dr Brendan Stubbs, a clinical psychologist, was interviewed. He referred to research into the psychological benefits of movement which suggests that moving around in your daily life is positive for your mind. In fact, some of his research in the area concluded that for people meeting the recommended guidelines of 150 minutes of activity per week, a person has a 30 per cent reduced risk of developing depression in the future.

If we combine movement with a focus on how you are moving, i.e. you are moving mindfully, then the benefits can become even greater because you are giving your mind a chance to rest from the everyday woes, and to focus solely on how you are moving. Oh, and if you add some deep breaths into that, then boom – bigger benefits still. This is because taking big breaths is a sure way of calming your nervous system (more on this in the breathing section, which can be found in Chapter 3).

Movement is Good For Your Memory

The World Health Organization reports that movement is great for "reducing cognitive decline, improving memory and boosting brain health". To elaborate a little, neuroscientists studying in this area have found a positive correlation between movement and the size of the hippocampus – the memory centre of the brain. This means that more movement can have a positive impact on your memory and also your creativity.

A WORD FROM
DR KATHARINE AYIVOR-NYGARD

Katharine (see page 209) knows a lot about the mind, being a clinical psychologist, and so I asked her to share her thoughts on how movement can benefit our wellbeing. Here is what she had to say:

"As a clinical psychologist, I have come to appreciate the importance of the connection between mind and body. It can be easy to focus on one and not the other, particularly when we are thinking about emotional and psychological wellbeing. However, what has become increasingly clear in recent research is the importance of various pathways in the brain and body that help us to regulate emotions and thus maintain overall management wellness.

One such pathway that has emerged as a potential reason for the link between certain activities and physical, emotional and cognitive wellness is the vagus nerve. It is the longest of the nerves that run from the brain to the body, running through organs in the neck, past the heart and to the abdomen. One of its functions is to balance our nervous systems.

One side (the parasympathetic side) reduces alertness, blood pressure, rate of breathing and heart rate, while the other side (the sympathetic side) does the opposite and increases alertness, heart rate, breathing rate and levels of energy.

This information is important to understand when thinking about how we can balance our nervous systems and impact our levels of stress, anxiety and fear. Our lives are increasingly busy and often stressful. Our brains and bodies are bombarded with signals that activate our fight, flight and freeze responses. While some level of stress is necessary to keep us motivated, too much of the stress hormones in our body has myriad negative effects.

Herein lies the beauty and power of practices such as Pilates and simple, mindful movements, which can involve deep breathing done in an intentional manner. This type of deep breathing enables the Vagus nerve to communicate with the diaphragm, which increases relaxation and in turn sends signals to the rest of our bodies and brains, with the overall impact being a more balanced nervous system and increased feelings of calm and wellbeing.

I am passionate about promoting the idea of holistic wellness; where we move away from the separation between brain and body. Learning to nurture and find ways in our daily lives to support both will stand us in good stead to meet the demands of daily life. When we develop regular movement practices, we invest time in our own health in so many important ways.

I find that sometimes when my clients are feeling stuck with intense difficulties, encouraging fundamental things such as regular movement, activities that are intentionally focused on deep breathing, can be a great step into empowering and increasing hope for change. On a personal note too, I have found that incorporating the practice of Pilates on a regular basis has boosted my feelings of wellbeing and mental clarity. I am a big fan!"

Why is Moving at Our Desks Good For Us?

As I mentioned in the introduction, I started Pilates At Your Desk after putting together a programme of simple movements for clients who would leave our lessons feeling amazing and then come back the next week with the same aches and pains. Yes, they would be doing their Pilates once a week, getting their steps in and going to various gym classes. But for the majority of the working day, they were staying still. So even though we could address the issues in class, the problems would creep back in because of their lack of varied movement in the period between classes. The programme of simple movements I put together was a hit, and there were fewer aches and pains all around (for those who did the moves, I should add!). Given this feedback, I decided to roll it out to more people.

It is quite simple really: the more you move in varied ways, the better you feel. Even if it is just a minute here and there intermittently throughout the day, it all adds up, and the great thing about this kind of movement is that you don't even have to leave your workspace to do it, and you certainly do not need to go and change your clothes. Integrating movement into our work routines in this way can be particularly important and beneficial given the amount of time we often spend in our workspaces.

Moving at your desk can help you to feel:

- Less stiff
- Less achy
- Longer/taller
- Stronger
- More mobile
- Calmer/more clear-headed
- More productive

- More balanced
- More coordinated
- Energized – and ready to do more movement
- Happier (it's difficult not to be!)

A WORD FROM
SARAH WOODHOUSE

I asked one of my mentors, Sarah Woodhouse (see page 208), movement expert and Pilates educator, for her thoughts on why movement at your desk is important. This is what she had to say:

"It is the case that 'motion is lotion'. All movement – fidgeting, wriggling, twisting around in your chair or dancing around it – is better than staying in the same position for long periods. The spine hates stillness. Even in the event that you could maintain great sitting posture, your spine and neck are going to thank you more if you move frequently."

So, I think we have set out a reasonable case for why we should all be moving more, and moving more at work specifically. But what about if our job requires us to sit or stand still for much of the time?

Case Study: Simone Reilly

Job role: Senior business partner (senior HR professional)

Number of hours spent sitting for work each day: 9–10

Number of movement breaks per day: 5–6

Time spent moving in working day: 1.5 hours! I try to move at least every hour and I walk my dog every lunchtime.

How do you move when at your desk? I follow the PAYD Instagram and use the short videos. I try to do regular shoulder circles, move my feet and my hands, move my neck from side to side and up and down. Oh, and I fidget a lot!

What reminds you to move? My smart watch buzzes every 30 minutes, or when I start to feel stiff.

How does more movement make you feel? More relaxed, less stiff, more focused – just generally better about myself.

Anything else that you would like to share? I try to squeeze the PAYD movements into my day when I can – waiting for my computer to turn on, while a document is loading, while watching a training video.

Case Study: Eloise McNeile

Job role: Community engagement strategist, tech

Number of hours spent sitting for work each day: 8

Number of movement breaks per day: 4–8 (every 45 mins or 2 hours if I have back-to-back meetings).

How do you move when at your desk? I tend to lift my legs against the wall of so that my legs are straight and feet are flat on the wall; I find that rather comfortable. Also, if I remember, I lift my arms up in the air and do little circles with my hands while I lower my arms. I also stand up to have a wiggle often.

What reminds you to move? Kerrie-Anne's Instagram account was my initial daily reminder. I look at my Instagram probably 4 times a day (eek!) so would see either one of Kerrie-Anne's posts or stories that would remind me ... and now it is just a habit, as though my body says, "Right, it's time to move."

How does more movement make you feel? It definitely makes a difference in my posture and my energy – I know when I have spent too much time at my desk, I feel much more lethargic at the end of the day.

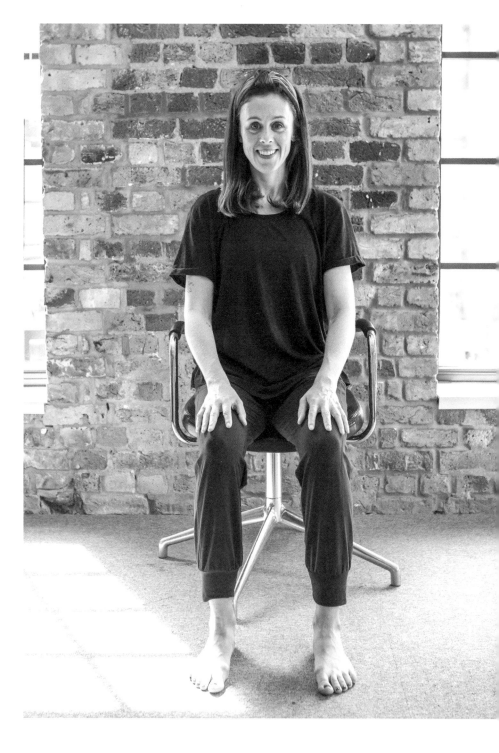

chapter 2.

Sitting and Standing

Thinking About How We Sit

In today's world, more jobs are geared toward sitting. It varies from person to person, of course, but many people with desk-based jobs may find themselves sitting for up to eight hours a day. And that is before you add on all the incidental sitting we do when we're eating, commuting, reading, watching TV and socialising.

I have already set out that movement is better for our bodies than lots of sitting, but what does this mean for someone who *has* to sit for work? Sitting in itself is not the concern. It is more that we tend to stay in our preferred seated position for long periods at a time, day after day. It requires little energy and often doesn't allow a balance between the two sides of the body. Sitting in a fixed position for hours on end can lead to weak and underused muscles, alongside some overworked ones, a low-energy brain and, ultimately, various aches and pains.

Noticing Our Sitting Tendencies

A helpful starting point when trying to sit in a more active and balanced way is to take note of how you sit normally. For example, do you cross one leg over the other? Do you slouch, sit up on one leg or straighten your legs out and cross them at the ankles?

While all of these are valid positions, there are some ways to sit that are more active (i.e. which get your muscles to work harder) and others that are not so energetic.

Take a look at the image opposite. This is what I would call "sitting like a croissant", where the bottom is tucked under and the top part of the back is rounded forward. There isn't much muscle "work" going

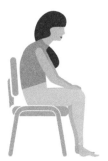
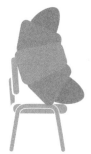

on. The legs are not active, the tummy muscles are switched off and you are potentially putting undue pressure on the lower back and the discs of the lower spine.

This croissant position is not only not very active, but it can also create a significant imbalance between the front and back of the body. I see lots of clients who come to me initially with lower back, neck and shoulder pain – and almost all have been sitting like this tasty little pastry.

WHEN WE CROSS OUR LEGS

Crossing your legs while sitting is perfectly valid. However, if we do it repeatedly and for long periods at a time, it can create imbalances between the right and left side of our body.

When we cross our legs, our leg bones are either turned in or turned out (internally or externally rotated) in our hip sockets. One side of our pelvis (the leg crossing side) is lifted higher than the other and our pelvis may also be slightly rotated. This can cause an imbalance at the back of the pelvis around the sacroiliac joint. If we do this for long periods of time, we may experience aches and pains around the hips, lower back and even further up the spine. Because it is also more difficult to sit up on your sit bones with a leg cross, we may end up slouching further up the body too.

HOW TO SIT IN A MORE ACTIVE AND BALANCED WAY

Active sitting involves consciously engaging some of your muscle groups. This could include those in your tummy, back or legs. If we can sit in a way that allows our bones to be stacked well, then this is going to be beneficial for your body. Here is one way of doing just that:

1. Have your feet flat on the floor, making sure your ankles are under your knees.

2. Keep your knees and feet pointing forward, rather than in or out.

3. Sit up on your sit bones (see opposite for a tip on finding these).

4. Your ribs should be over your pelvis (not lifted up to the ceiling).

5. Your shoulders should be down and wide (no squeezing together or rounding them forward).

6. Make sure your head is in line with your spine (one way to check in on this is to interlock your hands behind your head and push your head back into your palms).

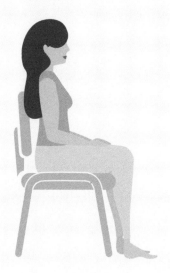

TIP: Your "sit bones" are located at the bottom of your pelvis. They are the two bones under your bottom: one on each side. When sitting up on them, you will have a right

angle where the back of your legs meets your torso on the chair. Another way to feel them is to roll up a small towel and sit up on it. You should feel your sit bones pressing down more easily in this position.

In this position you are using your core muscles (tummy and back) to hold you upright in a more vertical posture. If you are sitting equally on both sit bones, then you will be more balanced between the two sides of your body as well. You would not want to stay in this position for hours on end, either (remember: more movement is best). That said, a bit more of this and a little less of the alternatives is going to be kinder on the body and lends itself to fewer incidents of lower back issues and other aches and pains.

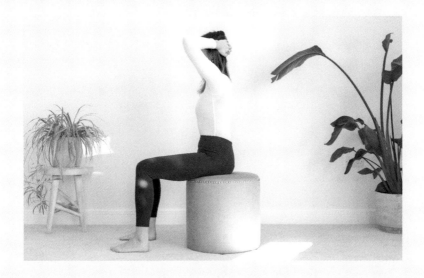

In practice, simply by introducing this way of sitting and mixing it up with your preferred way of sitting, you are already moving more just by switching between the two. Perhaps think of it like "a little bit of this and a little bit of that"!

TAKE AN INCREMENTAL APPROACH

Instead of trying to change the way you sit all day long, try taking an incremental approach to improving your sitting habits. For example, set yourself a target of sitting in the more active and balanced way described on page 44 for the first five minutes of each day. Over time, this can do two things:

1. You will create a new habit of sitting in this way; and

2. You will build the core strength to sit like this for longer.

As someone who used to sit with my legs crossed and with my back shaped like a croissant, I have definitely benefitted from sitting up in a more active and balanced way. My clients often tell me that sitting this way has been a "game changer", and that it has cured them of their back pain. Take my client Morag, for example, a retired NHS nurse. Here is what she found when she and her husband decided to "give up" leg-crossing ...

HOW MOVEMENT HELPS
MORAG ROSSI

"I started following Kerrie-Anne on Instagram during the first lockdown in 2020. I then joined her Zoom classes, normally twice weekly.

After the class ends, Kerrie-Anne is always happy to answer questions. On one occasion a fellow class-goer said her hip and bottom would feel great after class but would feel sore again the following week. Kerrie-Anne said that she noticed the lady in question would stand with one hip more forward than the other, and then asked if she crossed her legs often. Yes, she did, pretty much all the time at work. I listened to Kerrie-Anne explain the knock-on effects of hip mechanics on the pelvis and spine. It was a light bulb moment; from that day on, I made a concerted effort to uncross my legs! My husband decided to do the same, so we constantly 'ahem-ed' each other. Leg-crossing is now a thing of the past in our house and the habit is truly broken for us both. My hips and bottom muscles are much less tight now and I feel like I am much more balanced between the left and right side of my body and have also noticed a difference in how my shoulders are feeling too! Such a simple change that has made such a big difference to how we both feel."

(HYPER-)MOBILITY

There will be many of you out there who have the potential to move around quite a lot, and perhaps are capable of lots of movement at your joints. The extent to which joints are able to move with each other is described as mobility. Some of your joints will be more mobile than others, and you may be someone who is hyper-mobile at particular joints.

If so, it can be particularly important for you to check in on how you are sitting, as those of us who have a high level of mobility in our pelvis/lower back will often find it much easier and more attractive to embrace the croissant position. In fact, this may feel like the comfiest place on earth!

Taking time to sit up on your sit bones and having your pelvis in a neutral position can be particularly important for helping you to build strength in the muscles needed to support your bendiness.

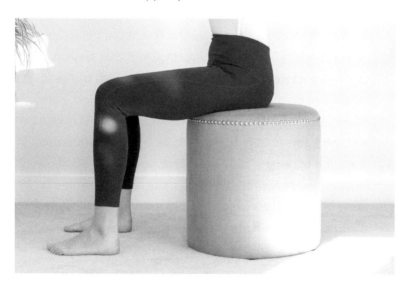

A WORD FROM
GRACE HURRY

I spoke to my exceptionally bendy friend, movement guru and ex-ballet dancer Grace Hurry (see page 208), about this issue, and here is what she said:

"It is a common misconception that being extremely flexible means being less at risk of aches and pain, and even injury.

When someone is hyper-mobile, their joints are generally less stable. Although they may have an impressive party trick up their sleeve, maintaining good posture for a hyper-mobile person can take just as much, if not more, work than someone who is inflexible. That's where sitting well comes in!

Sitting well can create a fantastic foundation for a hyper-mobile person. Practising a supported posture, especially when sitting for a long time, will help establish endurance and strength in muscles which will benefit all sorts of activities – even ones that don't involve a chair!"

What Should We Be Sitting On?

I often get asked about what to sit on and whether it is good to use a back rest or some other gadget. By all means, if this is what you have been advised to do by a medical practitioner, then please go ahead.

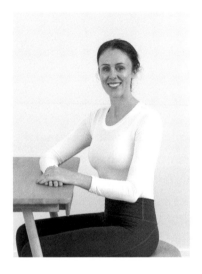 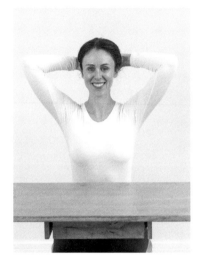

Personally, I choose to sit on a stool.

I just find that without a back rest, I have no option to collapse back onto it (the comfier it is, the more we will want to, even if this is not the best for our bodies). Not having a back rest means that when I start to feel a bit stiff, I do my moves while seated, or get up and walk around. I am not suggesting that back rests don't have a place, but if you do sit with one, then try to mix it up. Start at the front of your chair rather than relying on the back rest all day.

I also sit on the floor, up on my sit bones with my laptop propped up. When doing this I am constantly changing the position of my legs. I find that it is easier to sit this way when reading rather than typing because then I do not have to worry about what my arms are doing. This is a great way of sitting if you can comfortably sit up on your sit bones, otherwise you will need to pop something under your bottom so it is less demanding on the legs and hips. If you have tight hips, this may not be a comfortable option.

I have clients who sit on Swiss balls. These work well, as you can sit up on your sit bones and they add an extra stability challenge, so you are constantly moving a little to stay balanced. (Be aware that balls come in different sizes, so be sure to check which size works for your height before investing.)

I also recently tried wobble seat pads. I thought this was a rather ace way of getting you to sit on your sit bones while negotiating stability, so this gets a thumbs up from me too.

I have also, while writing this book, been alternating between standing and sitting and have been using a Harmoni desk (see page 207) which is excellent because it can be adjusted in height. I have set out on pages 53–9 some things to consider when you stand.

A WORD FROM
JULIE DRIVER

I thought I would invite my friend Julie Driver (see page 208), an excellent Pilates educator, horse whisperer and Pilates for equestrians expert, to speak about active sitting as someone who teaches people how to sit well on a horse. Here is what she had to say:

"Horse-riding is a sport, and although it is active, you cannot get away from the fact that most of the time the rider is sitting.

In fact, equestrianism is the perfect example of 'dynamic sitting': although a rider's posture may look static, it is constantly being challenged by the movement of the horse.

Before riding, I encourage my riders to mobilize their hips, move their backs, open their chests and work their shoulders with a short five-minute warm up. Even this small amount of movement can make a vast difference to their interaction with their horse and improve their seat in the saddle and their balance.

Imagine what a five-minute movement break can do for your day!"

What About Standing?

A regular question at Pilates At Your Desk workshops is whether we should all have standing desks. The research out there is mixed on this, but I think that mixing up standing and sitting to work is a good first step to being less sedentary. You use more energy to stand than you do to sit (although not as much as you would use when in motion), and alternating between sitting and standing may also be good for your mood. If you're in an after-lunch slump, simply standing up may give you a boost of energy. Doing a full-body wiggle would energize you even more!

How You Stand Matters

As was the case with sitting, how you stand – and the length of time that you remain in particular standing positions – matters. Repeatedly holding your body in a fixed position for long periods can give rise to aches and pains, irrespective of whether you are sitting or standing. This is certainly what I have observed with clients with standing jobs, such as healthcare workers or chefs.

Just as we did with sitting, therefore, a good first step is to notice your own standing tendencies, as this can help point to where change may be most beneficial.

So, how do you like to stand? Or, rather, how do you tend to end up standing when standing up for a sustained period of time?

One common tendency I come across a lot is leaning: forward and/or to one side. Here are some examples:

Stand on both heels!

A couple of years ago, I spent a few days at a London brewery working with groups of staff throughout the business (who had a mixture of sitting and standing jobs). What I found remarkable was that a number of the people with standing jobs who came to see me all experienced the same issue – lower back pain. When I explored the issue with them in more depth, I realised that all of these staff were wearing steel toe cap boots which, because of the sole of the shoes, tipped the weight of the person's feet to the front of the shoe (and therefore not on the heel).

To compensate for this (so they would not fall over), each person was also either pushing their pelvis forward or tucking it under while standing. This meant that the natural curves of the lower back were not being honoured.

As a way of helping with this, I suggested some heel connection exercises (see pages 54–5), as well as some guidance on how to stack your bones in a way that keeps things lengthened within the body (see pages 58–9).

A great way to immediately find more heel connection is to lift all of your toes (but keep the balls of your feet down). You will feel your weight transfer backward and your heels will, as a result, press into the floor more.

Yes, this was based on specific observations in the workplace, and of course other things could have contributed to this cohort's experience of lower back pain, such as the fact that they were bending a lot too (which is why we also worked on moving from the pelvis to bend – something we will get to later). But the fact is that addressing just one issue of potentially several had a positive impact. I checked in to see how people were doing on this front and the feedback was that the exercises had made a difference.

Don't be a leaner!

Not only can we shift our weight too far forward when we stand, but we can also stand more on one leg than the other (for many people who work at standing desks, this tends to be the side where the mouse is located). I remember teaching a client years ago who was excited to tell me about her new standing desk. She mentioned that she also had a niggle in her hip which she had previously experienced years earlier, but which had then disappeared until recently.

I noticed that her hip looked more compressed on her leg bone on that side. I asked her if she knew whether she leant on that leg. She said that she did not think so. During the lesson, we worked on moving that leg around in the hip socket and finding more length through her torso, while stretching out the mid-back and opposite shoulder. She found this to greatly improve how her hip felt.

At the end of the session, we chatted as she was leaving. As soon as she became settled in a standing position for the chat and began talking, she started leaning on said leg! It turned out to be tendency that – until that point – she had not consciously noticed.

WHAT CAN WE DO TO STAND IN A MORE ACTIVE AND BALANCED WAY?

When it comes to standing, I always tell my clients to try to make sure that their weight is evenly distributed over both feet.

It can be difficult to know when our weight is and isn't evenly distributed, however, so here are some specific aspects of standing that you can "check in" with in order to try to find a more balanced and active standing position.

TIP: Experiment with different types of footwear and going barefoot, as well as on different surfaces (carpet, floorboards, stone, etc.), as each will tend to give different levels and forms of feedback that it can be helpful to become more aware of.

Equal weight on both feet

Sway from side to side, shifting weight onto your left foot and then onto your right. Try to get both of your feet acquainted with the floor, and notice how the feeling differs when more and less weight is put on either side. Then try to adopt a position that spreads your weight evenly across both feet.

Equal weight at the front and back

Shift your weight onto the front of your feet (pressing onto the balls and toes), and then on to your heels. Do this a few times, and then try to stand with your weight distributed evenly over the front and back of your feet. Try to notice how this compares with how you might normally feel when standing, as this can help us understand less balanced ways that you may tend to settle into.

TIP: Using a mirror can be helpful here, as many of us may be surprised to find out how much we routinely tend to lean forward when standing.

Stand evenly on the insides and outsides of your feet

Roll your weight onto the inside and outside of each foot a few times. Try to notice how different positions compare to what you might normally do, i.e. where you tend to put more weight. After experimenting with how different ways of distributing your weight feels, try to stand evenly on both the insides and outsides of your feet.

Lift your arches

First, imagine your heels, the ball of your big toe and the ball of your little toe on each foot are being sucked into the floor. Try to keep the toes themselves relaxed – if you find yourself gripping your toes, try lifting all of your toes up and gently placing them down again (doing this a few times can help). When you have your weight settled, try lifting your arches up and away from the floor. They won't move far, but it can help your feet to be more engaged and active while standing.

The above steps should all help you stand evenly on and across both feet and – bonus – the very act of trying to find balance counts as movement! Now to the rest of your body ...

Stack your leg bones

Now check where your leg joints are. For each leg, you want the side of your hips (the widest part) to be over the side of your knees and your ankles, so all the bones are stacked on top of each other.

This can be a particularly good check for those of us who overuse our knees – that is, those of us who pull our knees right back, so the leg is shaped like the bow of a bow and arrow. This is an overly extended position for our knees to be in and can sometimes lead to excessive use of the knee joints. So, stacking our leg bones when we stand can help prevent this, and can also provide a handy reference point for those of us who are unsure when our legs are actually straight or not.

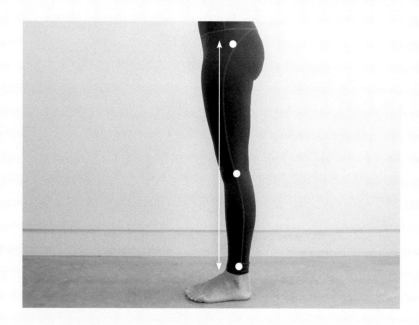

Keep your pelvis in "neutral"

As well as having your pelvis balanced over your leg bones, you want to make sure that your pelvis is in "neutral". That is, your pelvis should be in the same position that was described in the sitting section. Try to notice if you are tending to stick your bottom out, or tucking it under. It can be helpful to experiment by deliberately (but gently) sticking your bottom out and then tucking it under, before trying to settle in an intermediate position. (I have written more on this in Chapter 3 in the Pelvis section on pages 102–110.)

Below are some images of the pelvis in different positions. The first is in neutral; the second is tucked under; the third is sticking out. Stand side on in front of the mirror and see where your pelvis wants to live.

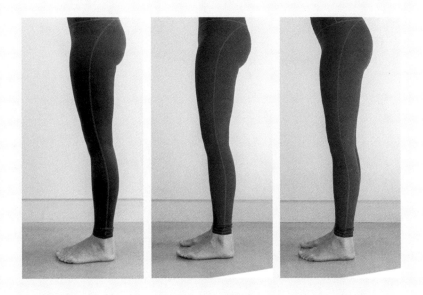

Take an Incremental Approach

As with sitting, try to take an incremental approach to changing your standing habits. Identifying some specific points in time when you can look to "reset" your standing position – making use of the above checklist – can be helpful. For example, when you first arrive at your workplace (if standing), and when you return there after breaks. You can then look to build up from there.

I have had a lot of clients with lower back pain see a massive reduction in this simply by being more conscious of where their pelvis is in space, including when standing. On page 62 is a story from Samuel, someone who experienced acute back pain for almost a year before changing how he stood and lining his bones up better! By simply addressing the way he was standing and by adding in more movement, his back pain reduced. We'll be talking more about the pelvis and bum gripping – which Samuel also refers to – later.

We have now established that:

- sitting can impact negatively on your health if you do it for long periods at a time

- mixing up sitting and standing is better (but you need to be mindful of how you do both)

- standing is more active than sitting

We have said throughout that movement is best and that we should do this often and keep it varied, so now let's get moving!

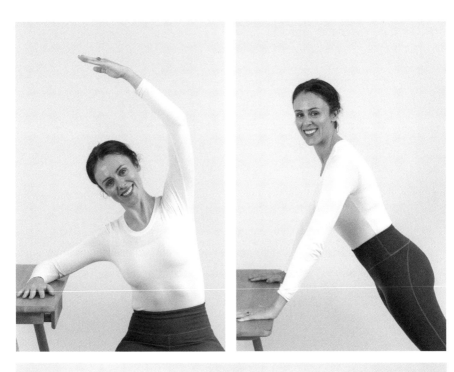

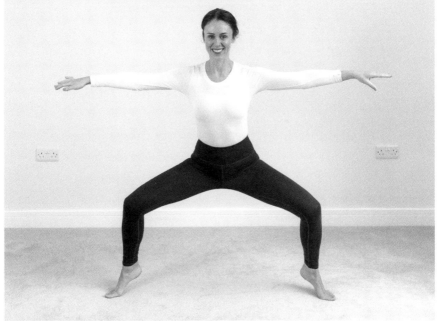

Case Study: Samuel Markusse

What pain were you experiencing? I had pain in my lower back and the right side of my bottom and leg. I was bending to the left when I stood, and couldn't walk for more than five minutes.

What did you find helped most from our work together? The most immediate change was that Kerrie-Anne helped me to stand well. She immediately noticed I gripped my bum whenever I stood up or tried to stand straight, and she helped me stand and relax these muscles. After explaining that I had a "sway back", where I push my pelvis forward, she taught me to push into my heels to bring my pelvis back.

I would hear Kerrie-Anne's voice in my head saying, "Don't be a bum gripper!" and "Push into the heels." The change was instant. Within a week, I could walk for 15 minutes without being in pain. A week later I was able to have a longer conversation with someone standing up. I felt so happy!

How you do feel now? So much better! Last weekend I walked for 3 hours with a toddler in my backpack and I felt fine! I feel looser and I definitely don't need surgery anymore. I feel relieved and hopeful that I will heal completely and that if my back plays up again, there's a way to get better.

Case Study: Dr Philippa Banahan

Job role: GP Partner

How long do you sit for each day? 11 hours when working

Number of movement breaks per day: 4–6 (short) movement breaks to get up where I can, but I move around on my seat a lot more than this.

Time spent moving around: 30 minutes of actively getting up between patients. The number will be more than this because I move at my desk.

How do you move when at your desk? I stand up when not with patients to walk. I am a big fan of spine stretches and generally moving my spine around.

What reminds you to move? Twinges of back pain make me move (terrible I know!) and feeling sluggish. Writing this has reminded me that I need to move more!

How does movement make you feel? More movement makes me feel more energized, relaxed and productive. I also feel much less back pain at the end of the day if I have moved around.

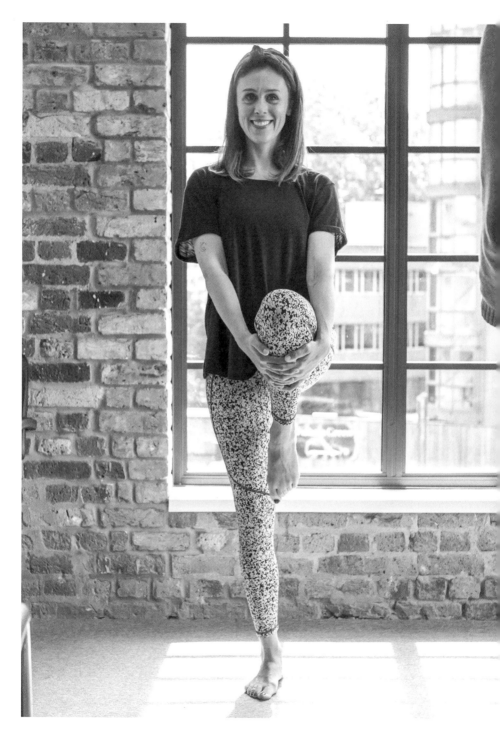

chapter 3.

The Move More Moves

We have now reached the juicy part of the story, where you get to learn the moves that you can do at your desk.

The movements in this chapter can be done seated or standing, and I would encourage you to think of them as a toolkit that you can pick and choose from whenever you need to move a particular body part. I have suggested that you do each movement a few times. To be more precise, I would suggest doing 6–8 repetitions. When you are doing one side at a time, do 3–4 repetitions on each side.

I will describe each of the moves in turn, as well as set out some "cues" that can provide helpful indicators and reminders of things to look out for. I'll also give you some suggested combinations of moves (let's call them routines), and ideas for how different moves can be incorporated into your working day – and made more incidental – are provided in later chapters.

Remember, the best type of movement is that which is **varied** and **frequent**.

You will notice that I speak mostly of bones when talking about the body parts to move. I do this for a couple of reasons:

- Firstly, there are far fewer bones in the body than there are muscles, making it easier to communicate what we are trying to achieve.

- Secondly, as there are usually lots of muscles working in one way or another when moving particular bones, it is often more difficult to visualize the exact location of the movement we are aiming for, so it can be easier, and more helpful, to talk about the bones.

I have provided images as well as written descriptions of each movement, which are intended to provide a base. Where helpful, I have shared more detail. These details are important as we often tend to fall back on favoured ways of moving, and the details and cues are intended to help us engage our bodies in different ways. Our bodies get used to moving certain parts over and over and many of the smaller, and deeper, muscles do not get so much action.

One aim of this section is to get you moving those "less up for it" parts more too. This is your chance to notice that even small movements – if done carefully – can be very effective. This is because the difficulty and effort comes not in, say, being able to lift our arms per se – many of us can find relatively easy ways of doing that – but rather in doing it in specific ways that bring other, less used, parts of our bodies into play. Doing this, and strengthening those more neglected muscles, can help save the more eager and "up for it" parts of our body from getting hurt!

None of this will come straight away, but if we can find different forms of engagement and notice how that feels, then it gives us something to try to come back to (and notice when we have moved away from).

Now for the moves, which – after a bit of warming up – are set out in the following pages by body parts/areas.

The shake break

Before describing movements geared toward specific body parts, I want to introduce you to one of my favourite ways to move. This is what I do at the start of every Pilates At Your Desk workshop, and something I probably do myself at least six times a day. It's very simple; you just stand up and shake all your body bits out. This is how I teach it:

1. **Start by shaking out your feet:** Lift your left foot off the floor and wiggle it around a little, point and flex your toes, and then replace it and do the same with the right.

2. **Move onto your legs:** Lift one leg out to the side and give it a little shake, and then do the same with the other. A little Irish jig-esque action with legs shaking out to the side would work. Or if you prefer, go for a full-on Hokey Cokey style!

3. **Wiggle your bottom:** Shake it à la Shakira (side to side – let it be free!).

4. **Jiggle your belly:** Wobble it around. A little bouncing helps with this.

5. **Shimmy your chest:** Get the shoulders involved too!

6. **Throw your arms in the air like you just don't care!:** Bring them above your head almost like you're swatting flies.

7. **Move your head around:** I like to embody the nodding-dog-in-a-car vibe when doing this, letting my head move freely!

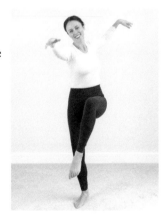

8. **Do all of the above all at once!** Really go for it. Get that heart rate up and make sure all those body parts are moving. Make yourself smile!

Shoulders and Chest

I always ask at the start of a workshop for a show of hands of people who have experienced shoulder aches at some point. Each time the majority of attendees raise a hand (and perhaps those who don't can't because of a sore shoulder!). The shoulders are a place where we can hold lots of tension. We overuse some parts and underuse others, and can experience aches in this area of our body because of how we position ourselves when working.

One key underlying issue is that there is often a mismatch between where/what we *think* the shoulder is, and where/what it *actually* is. This can mean that the top parts of our shoulders often get overused, because these are the areas we tend to think of using when we need to do something with our "shoulders". Given this, we can end up feeling tense and achy in this area.

With the shoulder movements described below we are trying to get the other parts of the shoulder gang to do their jobs, and give those poor guys at the top a well-earned tea break!

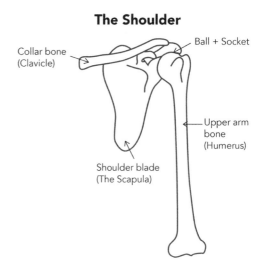

The Shoulder

Collar bone (Clavicle)

Ball + Socket

Upper arm bone (Humerus)

Shoulder blade (The Scapula)

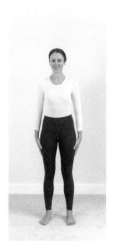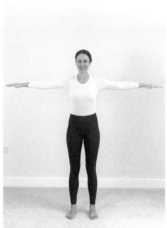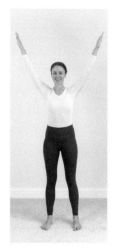

LIFTING YOUR ARMS ABOVE YOUR HEAD

There are a few routes you can take to get your arms over your head. Let us focus on the trajectory where you take your arms out to the side and up to your ears and look at what moves what:

- When your arms lift sideways from your hips to shoulder height, this is predominately your arm bones moving inside the shoulder socket.

- Once they go from shoulder to overhead, this becomes a job for the shoulder blades, which swing out to the side and up.

- When the arms return to chest height, the shoulder blades swing down and in, back to their start position.

- When you return your arms from chest height to your hips, this will be the arm bones moving in the socket again.

Try it without thinking and see which bit does the job in each step. Is it the tops of the shoulders by any chance? Now try again, but this time read the steps on the previous page as you go. See, I bet it made a difference. You're welcome, tired tops of shoulders!

For our shoulder blades to work efficiently and to prevent against injury, we want to be able to move these guys in all of the above ways. The movements on the next few pages explore how.

TYPING AND YOUR CHEST MUSCLES

It might surprise you to know that our chest muscles – the pectoralis muscles – are constantly being shortened as we work at a desk because of how we position our arms (forward of our bodies). This can mean we start to pull the shoulders forward and into a rounded position. Hello, slouchy shoulders! But it doesn't have to be this way.

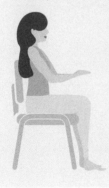

It is not really our fault that so much of our lives is geared toward having our arms forward of the body, and we can do something about it by taking the arms into different positions to stretch these muscles. See the next few pages for some ideas on this.

Elbows

Organizing where your elbows are can make a difference to how your shoulders and wrists feel when working. Some of us have very bendy elbows and can hyper-extend at the elbow joint when engaging in some movement (a similar issue can also arise for other joints, but elbows are particularly relevant here). This is commonly referred to as "locking" your elbows.

To check for this, bring your arms to chest height directly in front of you, palms facing down.

Do your elbow creases look up, or in? If up, the chances are you are locking them out. So, when your arms are out in front of you, have the creases looking in (toward each other) and not up.

When your arms are out to the side, the creases should look forward and not up.

When your arms are down by your side or overhead, elbow creases should look in.

Let's now turn to the movements.

THE MOVEMENTS

Lift and melt

This movement is great for easing tension around the tops of the shoulders as well as improving shoulder blade mobility.

1. Tap the back of your armpits with your hands. Then bring your arms to the sides of your hips to start the movement.

2. Take a big breath in, and as you do, push your shoulders up to your ears, moving from where you tapped.

3. As you breathe out, relax your shoulders down your back.

4. Do this a few times and see if you can melt those shoulders down more each time.

Shoulder circles

Like the previous exercise, this movement is great for easing tension around the tops of the shoulders and improving shoulder blade mobility.

1. Take a big breath in, and as you do, push your shoulders up to your ears, moving from where you tapped.

2. As you breathe out, squeeze your shoulder blades toward each other and roll your shoulders down your back.

3. After a few repetitions, change direction: squeeze your shoulder blades toward each other first. Push the shoulders up to your ears. Roll your shoulders forward and down your back.

Elbow circles

This movement is also great for shoulder mobility and a nice one for those with restricted mobility in the shoulder or chest area. My friend Carrie, a fellow movement teacher, recommends this as part of her work in post-operative breast cancer rehabilitative movement.

1. Place your fingertips onto the tops of your shoulders.

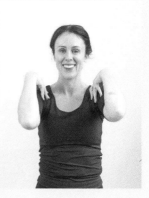

2. Draw big circles with your elbows, first forward, then backward.

Elbow swimming

This is great for shoulder mobility and tightness and upper back tightness.

1. Place your fingertips onto the tops of your shoulders.

2. Bring one elbow forward, up to your ears, and circle back behind you.

3. Repeat with the other elbow but at a lag – à la elbow backstroke.

4. Do a few of these with your chest facing forward, and then start to turn your head and upper back to look toward your back elbow, looking from left to right as your elbow change.

5. Now change direction so that it becomes more like elbow front crawl.

Lifting and lowering your arms

Have a sense of your arms being connected to your back for this one, and remember to move from your shoulder blades and not just the tops of the shoulders!

1. Start with your arms down by your hips, palms and elbow creases facing your hips.

2. Inhale and lift your arms up in front of you to chest height.

3. Exhale and raise your arms above your head so that you are framing your head with your arms. As your arms go up have a sense of the tops of your shoulders going down, so they don't go up to your ears.

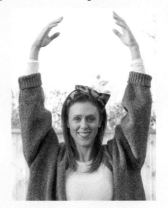

4. Return your hands to your hips on a full breath in and out.

Polishing the top of your halo

This is a great exercise that I picked up from my good friend Emma Bray. It's excellent for shoulder mobility and works the arms too! At the end, just let your arms hang down by your side for a bit. They will thank you for it.

1. Interlock your fingers and bring your arms in front of your chest, palms facing away from you.

2. Reach your arms above your head, palms facing up. (Remember: drop the tops of your shoulders away from your ears as your arms go up.)

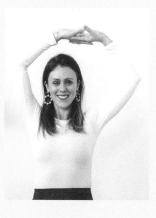

3. Bend your elbows out to the side.

4. Now, just like you're an angel polishing your halo (thanks for this analogy, Em!), start to circle your arms above your head, first one way, then the other.

TIP: Try to keep your torso still as you do this exercise, so you focus on moving from your shoulders.

Cactus arms

This movement is great for stretching the chest. It gets the shoulders moving and is good for arm strength and for working those upper back muscles too.

1. Straighten and lift your arms out to the sides of your body and in line with your shoulders with your palms facing forward.

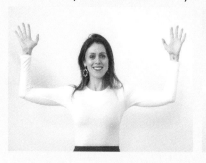
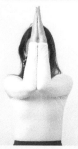

2. Bend at the elbows to make a right angle with the palms facing forward – a bit like a three-pronged cactus!

3. Bring your arms forward in front of you so that your palms touch. If your palms don't touch, don't worry! Just bring them as close together as you can.

4. Moving from the shoulder blades, i.e. pulling them toward each other, open your arms back out to the side.

The robot

This one is also great for shoulder mobility and strength, as well as arm and upper back strength.

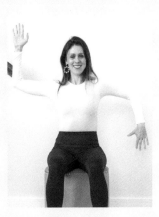

1. Straighten your arms out to each side so that they are in line with your shoulders.

2. Bend at the elbows to make a right angle with the palms facing forward.

3. Turn one arm down so your fingertips are now pointing to the ground, keeping the right angle at the elbow.

4. Switch arms – hello, robot!

Hug a tree

This is great for stretching the chest muscles and working the arms and shoulder muscles.

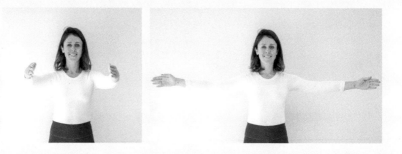

1. Bring your arms out straight in front of your chest.

2. Turn your palms and elbow creases to face inward with a micro-bend at the elbow – like you're hugging a medium-sized tree.

3. Pull your shoulder blades toward each other, opening your arms out to the side. (Now you're hugging a massive tree!)

4. Return your arms to the medium-tree hug.

Arm pulses

This is a lovely movement for stretching the chest and counteracting all that forward arm action. It's great for strengthening the arms too!

1. Lift your arms either side of you, bringing them up to shoulder height.

2. Make sure that they are in line with the front of your shoulders (i.e. not behind your body), palms face down.

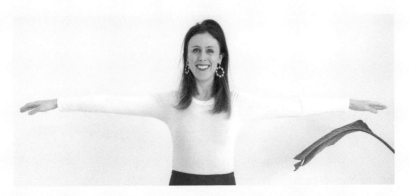

3. Relax the tops of your shoulders down away from your ears. Feel the back of your armpits engage. Sometimes I give the cue of imagining you're squeezing lemons under the back of your armpits. Perhaps this helps you?

4. Imagine your hands are in a tug of war, so they are as far away from each other as possible. (Keep checking on your elbows – and make sure they don't lock out.)

5. Pulse the arms back a little bit behind the body and then return them so they are in line with the front of your shoulders.

You can then do the same thing with the palms facing up, backward and forward. In each case, remember to focus on pulsing the arms back.

TIP: At the end of every exercise, have a little wiggle to finish it off and get in a few extra seconds of movement. Especially where you have been keeping your spine still, a little wiggle of the spine will be well-deserved and is a good way of thanking it for being so stable.

Bonus Moves

Sarah Woodhouse (see page 208) has so many excellent feel-good moves up her sleeve, and here are two of her favourites, which you can do seated or standing.

The mighty yawn

1. Wrap your arms around yourself in a big hug and twist from side to side.

2. Inhale and peel your arms up over your head as if you are peeling off a sweater. Reach one arm then the other even higher a few times to stretch one side of your waist and then the other.

3. Exhale and circle your arms open and around behind you in the biggest circle you can to stretch your shoulders and chest.

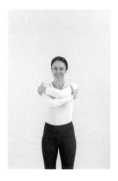 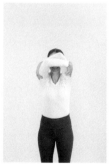 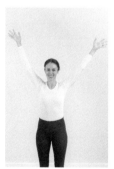

Swimming strokes vertically!

Start small and slowly make each stroke as big and stretchy as feels good. Hopefully these movements are already familiar. Together they are a great overall movement for your spine, neck and shoulders.

- **Backstroke:** With your pelvis facing forward, circle one arm backward and then the other. Move your spine as well as your arms. Look over your shoulder as you circle your arms. Make the biggest circles you can.

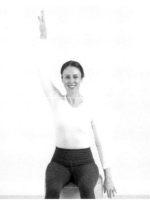

- **Front crawl:** With your pelvis facing forward, circle one arm forward, then the other. Reach across your body with your arm and allow your spine to curve forward.

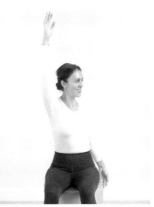

- **Breaststroke:** Palms down and/or palms up, perform breast stroke arms with your arms at chest height. If it feels good, lift your chest to the ceiling as your arms move to the sides and back.

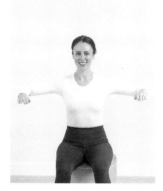

- **Butterfly:** Circle your arms around over your head from the back to the front, making the biggest circles you can with relaxed shoulders.

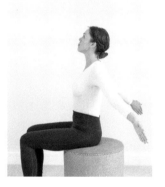

Neck

The head is heavy business, with the average adult human head weighing around 5kg (11lb). (For context, most newborn babies weigh less than that!) So, your neck has a real job keeping that head upright. Therefore, it is unsurprising that you can overuse your neck.

Your neck muscles and the joints in this part of the body allow you to nod your head, turn it left and right, circle and tilt from side to side. We might look from side to side when crossing the road, or over your shoulder when in the car, but if you are sitting looking at a computer for hours each day, then the chances are, you are looking forward, and because the head is heavy, the weight of it pulls it forward and down.

You may have heard of terms like "text neck" or "tech neck". Well, there is a lot of discussion among movement practitioners as to whether our handheld devices are responsible for neck pain. As with many things, you can find studies that argue either way.

However, there's no denying that looking down at your phone or laptop for long periods at a time is going to impact you. It will cause muscle imbalances between the front and back of your upper body, and over time this can impact your head and neck positioning. For some people this is pain-free, but for others this can cause tension and pain. The movements in this section will keep your neck moving, strong and in good alignment.

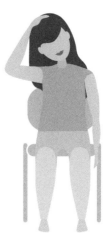

HELPING YOUR NECK AT WORK

Have devices at eye height

Set your computer at eye height. If you have a laptop, you can get a stand and freestanding keyboard. Hold your phone at eye height too. If you don't think you can remember this, you could set your screensaver as a reminder – "I like to be at eye height".

Nod from your ears

Many of us overuse the base of our neck as we look down from here. Another place to look down from is actually at the ears. Try it! Pop your index fingers next to the entrance to your ears and nod your head from there. It may feel weird, but it will give you a nice 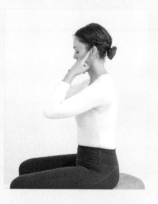 neck stretch. Remove your fingers and see if you can look down by moving from your ears, rather than the base of your neck.

Jaw clencher

If you are someone who clenches their jaw when concentrating, I suggest sticking Post-its around your working area to remind you to relax your face, as it adds to tension in the neck. Gentle face massage[12] is great for this too. If you clench at night, a quick massage before bed and first thing in the morning will help.

THE MOVEMENTS

Head and neck alignment

This movement is great for working the top of those back muscles and reminding you of where your head is in space. I do this often because I spend a lot of time looking down (mostly at pelvises and other body parts).

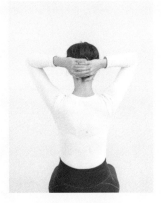

1. Interlock your fingers and place your hands behind your head, thumbs on the soft bits under your skull.

2. Breathe in and press your head and hands into each other. You should feel the muscles at the top of your spine working.

3. Breathe out and feel your ribs moving toward your belly button as you continue to press your head back.

4. Breathe in and out to relax your head and give it a wiggle.

Head circles with eyes

This is a lovely one for working through any neck tension, and it also gives your eyes a break from the screen.

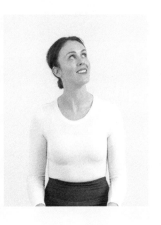

1. Imagine you have a pen on your nose. Draw a small circle with the pen, going slowly.

2. Also draw the circle with your eyes.

3. Gradually increase the size of the circle.

4. Once you have done 6 circles, go the other way, starting small and increasing in size.

Turning your head

1. Imagine your chin is on a cake stand and as you turn it left and right, it stays on one level (it does not go up or down).

2. Breathe in, look to the right and then turn your head right.

3. As you breathe out, bring your head back to the centre.

4. Repeat on the other side.

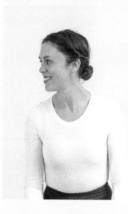

Front-of-neck stretch

1. Lower your shoulders as far away from your ears as possible, reaching your arms down toward the floor.

2. Take your right ear to your right shoulder (not shoulder to ear!) and keep your gaze forward. You should feel a lovely stretch down the left side of your neck.

3. To increase the stretch, take your right hand and place it under your left collar bone. Gently pull down.

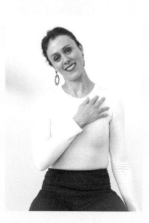

4. Then, open your mouth and drop it toward your right shoulder. This will relax your jaw and increasing the stretch further.

5. Repeat for the left side and feel the tension melt away!

Pez[13] head

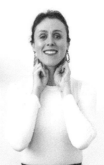

This is one of my favourite movements to teach, mostly because I like saying, "It's time to get your Pez head on!" (It makes me chuckle, if no one else!). It's brilliant for releasing jaw and neck tension too.

1. Take your middle finger and your index finger and place them on the soft part under your ear and just before your jawbone.

2. Press up a little, open your mouth, and then start to nod your head up and down (that's the Pez head part – minus the sweets).

3. Do this a few times.

4. You can then move your head from left and right, giving the jaw a massage as the jaw passes over your fingers.

5. It's nice to also draw circles with your head here, or maybe the odd infinity sign too.

6. Once you're finished, place your hands flat on your face and slowly open and close your mouth a couple of times, taking in big breaths as you go. It should feel lovely.

Spine

"A man is as young as his spinal column."
Joseph Pilates

If I had a pound for every time I heard someone say, "I've got a bad back, but it's just because I am getting old," I would be a very rich lady indeed.

There is a belief in western society that aches and pains are a sign of age, and that we are just to accept this as being the case. However, many of my clients, who range from the ages of 25 to 75, come to me with back pain – and in some cases, quite painful back issues, such as herniated discs and spondylolisthesis – and none of these clients now have daily back pain. Indeed, the biggest feedback I get from those who come to PAYD workshops, or who follow along on Instagram and do these moves, is that their back pain is much better (if not gone).

So, why is back pain so common?

Well, first of all, there is a lot going on back there, which means that it is a big area with room for system error. Our spine is made up of 24 bones: seven at the top (cervical spine), twelve in the middle (thoracic spine) and five at the bottom (lumbar spine).

Over the middle part you have your ribs and below the bottom part of your spine is your pelvis. Quite often we overuse our lower backs instead of moving the thoracic and the pelvis, and as a result these parts can become quite stuck. When the lower back does the job of the other parts on a repetitive basis, it can become overworked, tired and hurt. This can be on a muscular level, or indeed on a more serious level when it affects our discs (the cushion-like ligaments between each bone of the spine) and other structural systems.

There are ways to mitigate lower back pain by teaching the parts that do not move very much to move more, and also to keep all parts of the spine moving in the directions it is able to. The spine can bend side to side (side-bending); it can turn to face more left and right (rotation); it can bend forward (flexion); and it can bend backward (extension). Different parts of the back are better at doing different movements, e.g. the middle part of our spine, which naturally curves forward (kyphosis), finds it easier to flex than it does to extend, and conversely the bottom part, which naturally curves in, finds it easier to extend. This means that when doing our movements, we want to focus on getting the parts to do what they don't naturally do, so as to balance it out and not to be too flexed in the top and too extended in the bottom.

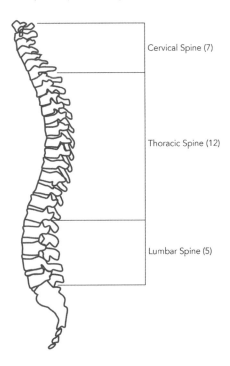

Cervical Spine (7)

Thoracic Spine (12)

Lumbar Spine (5)

Later on in the book, I will look at getting the pelvis and using breath to get the thoracic middle back to show up more for work, and there will be some combinations that look at tackling lower back tightness specifically. However, for now, we will focus on good movements that get the spine moving.

FLEXION

You may wonder why I suggest that sitting like a croissant is not a good idea and then talk about flexing your spine in the following exercises. It is true that sitting like a croissant does involve spinal flexion, but the devil is in the detail.

The difference is the journey to flexion. In the croissant scenario, the body is likely slumped and the spine is compressed. The flexion described in the following movements is one where you lengthen the spine to flex it. You engage the front of your torso to help you find a nice, long, even curve of the spine. The spine is decompressed as you increase the distance between your sit bones and the top of your head.

That said, I would not advocate you sitting in lengthened spinal flexion for long periods. It is good to keep the spine moving in all the directions it can, as well as keeping it in neutral.

THE MOVEMENTS

Side-bend

A side-bend – that is stretching the side of your body – is excellent for lengthening and strengthening your torso and creating more space for you to breathe. When doing this exercise, you want to try to keep both sides of the waist nice and long, so lifting your body up and over and not compressing onto the side you bend forward. I sometimes think it helps to imagine you are trying to reach your head to the ceiling the whole time, even when going over at the diagonal.

1. Sit on your sit bones with your hands interlocked behind your head.

2. Breathe in and side-bend over to the right. Keep your left sit bone down.

3. Breathe out to return to centre.

4. Repeat on the left side, keeping your right sit bone down this time.

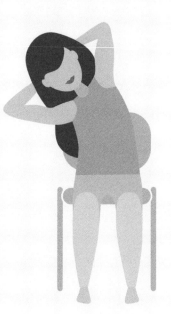

Side-bend with arms over head

This one is nice for getting the stretch all the way under the armpits. You may be surprised by how tight that area is when you first do it, so go with care.

1. Reach your arms above your head and grab your left wrist with your right hand. Drop the tops of your shoulders away from your ears.

2. Breathe in and side-bend over to the right, lifting your body up and over, keeping the body long on both sides of the waist (i.e. not compressing onto the right side). Remember to keep your left sit bone down.

3. Gently pull on the left arm to increase the stretch as your go up and over.

4. Breathe out to return to centre.

5. Switch wrists. Go to the other side, keeping your right sit bone down this time, gently pulling on the right wrist this time.

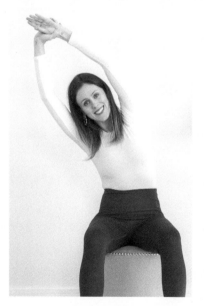

Rotation

I am a big fan of rotation because it feels good, it's useful in everyday life, it moves your spine and works your belly at the same time.

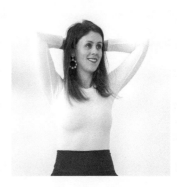

1. Sit on your sit bones with your hands behind your head.

2. Imagine your ribs are on a cake stand (as well as your chin (see page 86) – think of it as a two-tiered cake stand!). As you move left and right, the ribs stay on one level rather than going up and down.

TIP: *Do it in front of a mirror the first time if you can't feel this!*

3. Breathe in and rotate your spine to the right. Just your spine; don't move your pelvis for this one. Keep your hip bones facing forward.

4. Breathe out to return to centre.

5. Repeat on the other side, keeping those ribs on one level and your hip bones facing forward.

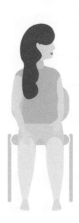

Rotate with hands on knees

I like this version as it gives you the added head rotation too.

1. Sit on your sit bones and put your hands on your knees.

2. Breathe in and turn your head to look right, then your shoulders, then your mid back, and lastly your lower back (but keep your pelvis still; your legs should not move).

3. Your right hand will glide up your leg.

4. Breathe out to return to centre.

5. Repeat on the other side. Head, shoulders, mid-back and lower back to left (so difficult to not say, "head, shoulders, knees and toes" here!).

Rotation with legs and arms in a "V"

This movement is the perfect antidote to how we are positioned to work, because it really opens the chest, works the top of the back muscles and makes you feel long and wide. I would suggest doing some side-bending, shoulders and other rotation first to make the most of it. It will feel challenging, but hopefully you will feel really stretched out after doing it.

1. Wiggle your bottom to the edge of your chair and bring your legs to a "V" shape. Press your heels into the floor and pull your toes back toward you.

2. Reach your arms up above your head into a "V" shape with your palms facing forward. Drop the tops of your shoulders down and away from your ears.

3. Palms facing forward, press your arms back as much as you can without your ribs thrusting forward.

4. Now it's time to imagine your ribs are on a cake stand (as well as your chin (see page 86) – that two-tiered cake stand again). As you move left and right, the ribs stay on one level rather than going up and down.

5. Breathe in and rotate your spine to the right. Just your spine; don't move your pelvis for this one.

6. Breathe out to return to centre.

7. Repeat on the other side, keeping those ribs on one level.

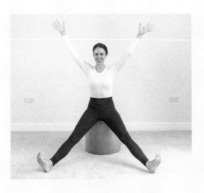
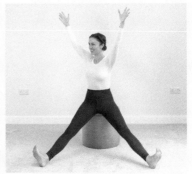
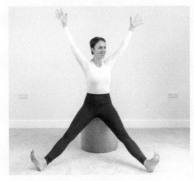

Flex your spine from bottom to top

This is a great movement for stretching the back while strengthening the tummy muscles. To get the most from it, we need to be quite precise about starting this movement from the sit bones, rather than the lower back, as we want to try to get the part that does not move as easily to give the more moving part a bit of a break.

1. Start by sitting up on your sit bones. You can have your hands behind your head for this movement too.

2. Breathe in and feel yourself getting taller (I like to imagine a tug of war between the sit bones and my head).

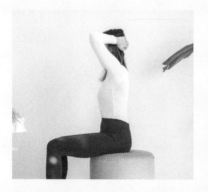 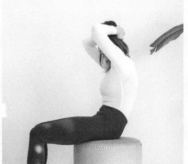

3. Breathe out and gently pull your belly button in toward your spine. At the same time, tilt your pelvis, starting at your sit bones and rolling to the back of your sit bones, toward your tail bone.

4. Keep pressing your head back into your hands as this will keep the spine in a lengthened curve and sequentially curve your back body from pelvis to head. Your body will form a C-shape.

5. Inhale to return to your start position, making sure to do this and every other step nice and slowly.

TIP: Take an extra inhale once you've reached your C-shape and draw your chest, ribs and belly toward your spine on the exhale. This will stretch your back more, getting more out of the exercise.

Extend the upper spine – lift collar bones

This particular movement is the opposite of the position we most often find ourselves in when working at a computer. It brings the head back into line with the spine by working the upper back muscles and playing with where your eye focus is, and it gently stretches the chest.

The lower back structurally bends this way, and so when doing this movement we want to really focus on moving from the upper back, otherwise the lower back will just jump straight in and do the work for us and we won't get as much out of the movement. So, again, we want to be precise about where this movement starts.

1. Start by sitting up on your sit bones. You can have your hands down by your sides or behind your head.

2. Imagine you're a puppet with strings attached to your collar bones. A puppeteer gentle pulls those strings, lifting your collar bones to the ceiling as you breathe in.

3. Breathe out and visualize your ribs dropping in toward each other and down to your hips as you continue to look up. If your hands are behind your head, keep pressing your head into your hands.

4. Breathe in and out to return to your start position.

TIP: If, like me, you have a ribcage that loves to lift up, then you might find that when you do this extension you just move your ribs, rather than extending from higher up your back. What I would suggest is putting one hand on your collar bones and the other on your bottom front ribs. As you do the extension, check that the lift comes from the collar bones rather than the ribs, otherwise it's another case of just moving the already moving parts more.

Cat/Cow

This exercise is taken from the mat and is commonly recognized as a yoga pose. I have translated it to sitting but kept the name because I like it. It is essentially a combination of the previous two movements, but makes use of both the top and bottom of the back at the same time (middle too!).

1. Start by sitting up on your sit bones. You can have your hands on your knees for this one.

2. Breathe in and grow taller, pressing your sit bones down and lifting the crown of your head to the ceiling.

3. For CAT: As you breathe out, gently pull your belly button in toward your spine and at the same time, tilt your pelvis from the sit bones, rolling to the back of your sit bones toward your tail bone.

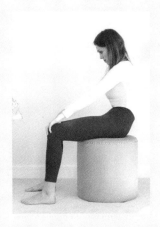

4. As with the lengthened flexion on page 97, sequentially curve the entire spine until your spine and head resemble a C-shape.

5. Breathe in, and on the exhale see if you can increase the back curve by tilting your pelvis a little more and pulling your belly button, ribs and chest into your spine.

6. Breathe in and out to return to vertical.

7. For COW: As you breathe in, start to tilt your pelvis the other way, sticking your bottom out and at the same time, lift your collar bones up to the ceiling.

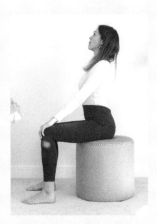

8. Breathe out and visualize your ribs dropping in toward each other and down to your hips as you continue to look up.

9. Breathe in and out to return to vertical.

Back flop

This is a lovely, calming rest pose that stretches your back and is a less severe option for people who cannot roll down to touch their toes from standing.

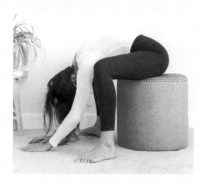

1. Start by sitting up on your sit bones. You can have your hands on your knees for this.

2. Breathe in to grow tall – imagine a hand on the top of your head and you are pressing up into it.

3. Breathe out, gently pull in the belly button and walk your hands down your legs. Your head and spine will follow until your hands reach the floor. Your head should end up dangling between your arms.

4. Take a few breaths in and out here, and feel free to sway from side to side if it feels nice.

5. Take a breath in. Breathe out to pull the belly up and roll your pelvis back to vertical as you walk your hands back up your legs to your start position.

Star and ball

This is one of my favourite movements ever and the one that I always use at the end of workshops. It's great for getting the energy up and is sure to bring a smile to your face. The star is a form of power-posing, so brilliant to do before a meeting. It gets your spine moving, your shoulders moving and is just an all over body experience. You can even speed it up to make it more of a cardio workout too.

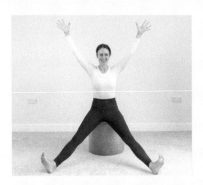 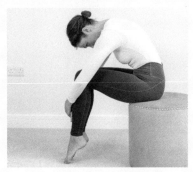

1. Start by sitting on the edge of your chair, up on your sit bones.

2. Bring your legs out to a "V" and do the same with your arms, so they are above your head. (You should look like a big star!).

3. Pull your legs together and bend them. Bring your hands to the front of your legs, rounding your back and bringing your head toward your knees. You should have formed a ball shape.

4. Alternate between being a big star and a little ball. I like to flex my feet when I am a star and point my feet as a ball. Give it a whirl and see how it feels.

Pelvis and Legs

Your pelvis – home of the derrière – sits between your spine and your legs. It is a pretty complicated structure with all sorts of things going on.

Your pelvis is bowl-shaped with effectively two sides (the hip bones) brought together at the sacroiliac joints. The sit bones (which I bang on about all the time) are at the bottom of the pelvis. Your upper leg bones slot into the side of each hip bone at a ball and socket joint.

There are lots of things that can happen at the pelvis and legs. For a start, your pelvis (with the help of all the muscles in this area) can move in different ways.

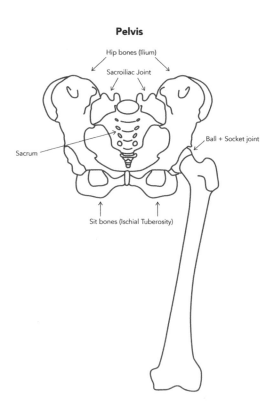

Pelvis

Hip bones (Ilium)

Sacroiliac Joint

Ball + Socket joint

Sacrum

Sit bones (Ischial Tuberosity)

In addition, the two sides of the pelvis can do different things. One side could be higher than the other (i.e. the front of the hip bone on one side is closer to the armpit on the same side) – known as a hip hitch. One side could also be more forward than the other – known as a rotation. With the latter, one way of telling is if one of your feet is more forward than the other when you are standing still.

*TIP: **Why not stand up now, wiggle around then stand still and see where your pelvis likes to live?***

Then we need to look at how your legs move with the pelvis. From the hip socket, legs can move forward, backward, out to the side, across the body; they also turn out and turn in. Legs can be bent at the knee too.

There are lots of muscles in this area that are responsible for moving your pelvis and legs, including:

- The gluteus muscles (your bottom muscles)
- The quadriceps (front of thighs)
- The hamstrings (back of thighs)
- The adductors (inside thighs)
- The abductors (outside thighs)
- The lower leg muscles

Like with other parts of the body, some muscles will do more work than others. The balance of effort can mean that other parts do not do as much and can be underworked. How we position our bodies when in a stationary position plays into this, as well as how we move.

Are You a Bum-Gripper?

I see a lot of clients who have a habit of gripping the sides of their bottoms, either because it helps with lower back pain, makes their bottom look smaller or because that's how they think they are supposed to make their bottom muscles work. For some, it's just how they've always stood.

Whatever the reasoning, bum-gripping has the effect of pushing the pelvis forward, a bit like in photos 1 and 2 opposite. The effect can be that some muscles (including those at the side of the bottom) work too much, while other parts of the glutes and the hamstrings get underused. Bottom-gripping can lead to pain in the lower back, hips, bottom and in other parts of the body.

So, as much as possible, we want that bottom to be free from the grip when we are going about our day to day, much in the same way that you would not constantly (and consciously) pull your shoulders up to your ears all the time.

Indeed, this sort of patterning can affect how we sit/stand (although it is a bit of a "chicken and egg" scenario, as how we stand/sit can affect which muscles work more than others!). So, let's explore this by looking at the position of the pelvis when we are standing.

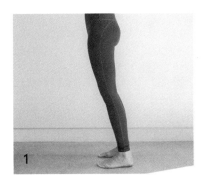 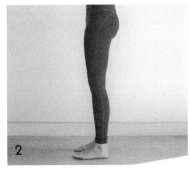

Photo 1: Here, the pelvis is pushed forward. This is more commonly known as a "sway back". The lower back is compressed.

Photo 2: Here, the pelvis is in a posterior tilt, such that the lower back curve is flattened out, and the bottom is tucked under.

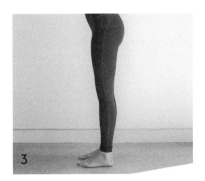 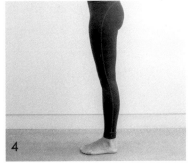

Photo 3: Here, the pelvis is in an anterior tilt. The lower back curve is exaggerated.

Photo 4: Here, the pelvis is in a neutral position, i.e. the natural curve of the back is not flattened or exaggerated. The side of the hip is stacked over the side of the knee and over the side ankle bone.

Where we hold our pelvis in space is important for what happens elsewhere in the body. Ideally, out of all the images on page 105, you want the pelvis to be in the position shown in the last one. Here, the natural curves of the spine are being honoured and the lower back is not being flattened or compressed in the way that it is in the other images.

People will come to me a lot with lower back pain, and quite often just addressing how they hold their pelvis in space helps massively to reduce their discomfort. This is not to say that we should keep the pelvis still and in neutral the whole time. Indeed, as with everything, movement is key. However, when being still, how we position our pelvis can make a massive difference to how our bodies feel.

If we translate this to sitting, a neutral pelvis is one where – surprise, surprise – the sit bones are pressing down. Sitting on your sit bones means less lower back compression and it helps to stack the rest of your body more effortlessly.

A WORD FROM
SARAH WILLIAMS

Here are some words from Sarah Williams, an NHS ward manager and paediatric nurse on a patient unit, whom I have taught for a few years now.

"As a nurse I had suffered with chronic back pain for about ten years, and when I started Pilates with Kerrie-Anne, that almost disappeared. Pilates is not something you do just for your lesson; it has changed the way I move throughout my day-to-day living. It has been the simple changes that have made the biggest difference: standing on my heels, sitting on my sit bones and breathing properly.

A big one for me has been how I position my pelvis when standing (and with my job I do a lot of standing). I did not realize that I constantly tucked my bottom under, gripping my bottom muscles and compressing my lower back. Introducing 'shake breaks' (see pages 67) into my routine, wiggling my bottom and making sure I stand on my heels have all helped me to stop doing this – and my back pain has disappeared!"

Differentiating Between the Pelvis, Lower Back and Legs

If your pelvis does not move as much as it could, then other body parts get involved more than they should to enable you to do certain movements. This applies to your lower back, which can end up doing lots of extra work because your pelvis is not up to the job (yet!). For many people, this contributes to aches and pains in the lower back region.

By focusing on movements of the pelvis, we can change this dynamic, thereby getting the pelvis more involved and taking the pressure off the lower back (quite literally!).

Our legs play a role in this too. Your legs meet the pelvis on each side at a ball and socket joint. This means that your leg bones have the potential to move in a full circular motion, much like the arms. It is important for hip health to keep the legs moving in the different ways they are able to. What can happen is that our legs can get stuck and only move in certain ways, and perhaps not as independently as they could. So, when you move your legs, your pelvis moves too. This can put pressure on the sacroiliac joint (sometimes one side more than the other), which can be another reason why we may feel back pain.

Pelvic Stability

Following on from this, the other element we need to consider is strength. The pelvis really is the anchor for your spine, and we want this to be a sturdy base. Yes, movement is great, but excessive movement around the joints of the pelvis can lead to too much instability around the spine. This is why we want the muscles in this area to be strong, but also to be working in an even, balanced way on both sides (left and right).

Being even on both legs helps stability around the pelvis. You can also strengthen your legs at the front, back, inside and outside in a balanced way to help with stability. A common issue I see is that many of us have strong front of thighs but not so strong hamstrings, and/or strong outside legs rather than inside. Part of what we will do in this section is try to make that distribution of strength more even.

SCIATICA

Sciatica is a pain in the bottom and/or legs caused by a pinching/ compression of the sciatic nerve, and back in my economist days and while pregnant, I experienced it down both legs. It is quite painful, and it is definitely distracting when trying to work. Over the years I have helped many clients overcome sciatica.

One thing I often hear is that sciatic pain is just a sign of getting old. Well, let me tell you: it is not.

In fact, it is most likely to be a compression of the lower back, which, in many cases, can be alleviated by better alignment of the pelvis and lower back, as well as – you guessed it! – more movement.

My personal experience of sciatica started when carrying a laptop on my shoulder on the train commute from Birmingham to London for work. Having one side laden with stuff meant that I was massively leaning on one hip. Add in a little hip rotation and a massive bum grip and boom – pressure on the sacroiliac joint and compression of the lower back. Man, that hurt.

My top tips for sciatica sufferers are:

- Make sure you stand/sit with your pelvis in neutral (no bum-gripping)

- Do not be a leaner

- Do movements which move the pelvis (hello, hip hinge) and the legs independently of the pelvis

- Move around lots (quelle surprise!)

- See a medical practitioner and a movement practitioner if you need extra help

To summarize, just like with other parts of our bodies, we need to move our pelvis and legs in a way that promotes balanced muscles, making them stronger and more flexible, as well as improving stability and mobility.

HOW MOVEMENT HELPS
LISA DAVIS

"For me, it is having my feet flat on the floor and having an awareness of the ball of my big toes when I am sitting is a game-changer. I have had to work hard to correct my constant knee crossing and shifting my weight over to one side of my hip (which was a nightmare because I had constant hip pain). I do this by sticking loads of Post-its around my screen! It definitely makes me feel more aligned and my hips are thankful."

THE MOVEMENTS

The march

This is just a great way of getting the legs to move without having to leave your seat.

1. Sit up on your sit bones with your feet flat on the floor.

2. Begin to march on the spot, being mindful that you stay even on both sit bones (there is that stability angle I was taking about).

TIP: *You could do it for a minute or two, speeding up the march to a seated jog/prance if you fancy! Just try to stay even on both sit bones so it is definitely a movement of the legs and not the hips too.*

The bottom shuffle

Yes, just like babies do, but on a chair rather than the floor. I like it because it challenges the hips to work unilaterally, gets your waist working and strengthens the pelvic floor. If you have a chair on wheels, you will want to secure it before trying this one.

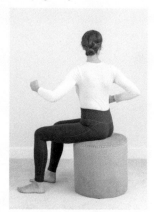

1. Start by sitting at the back of your seat, up on both sit bones.

2. Shuffle forward with one sit bone (so one side of the pelvis is more forward than the other).

3. Shuffle the other to meet it.

4. Keep going until you get to the front of your chair.

5. Now repeat the process, going backward this time.

Hamstrings and inside thighs

This is a very simple but effective way of strengthening these two areas, and it is one you could do while on a video call. This is also a great one for training your brain to connect your heels and should help with that heel connection when moving around on your feet.

1. While sitting, bring your legs together, or as close together as possible (if they do not come together, you could put a pillow between your knees).

2. Inhale, lift your toes and press into your heels.

3. Exhale and relax.

4. Inhale, and squeeze your inside thighs together (squeeze the pillow if you have that).

5. Exhale and relax.

6. Inhale, and do steps 2 and 4 together (heels and inside thighs).

7. Exhale and relax.

8. Repeat steps 6 and 7.

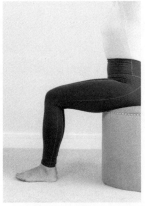

Hip hinge

In the hip hinge, we move our pelvis on our leg bones while they stay still. Our spine follows, going along for the ride. We do not change the curve of our lower back for this one – it's a movement of the pelvis and not a back bend.

This is a great exercise for realigning the pelvis and bringing awareness to the fact that our pelvis can move in this way. It is a fantastic stretch for the muscles which attach around the sit bones, and it helps to balance the two sides too. I also love this as a way of helping clients who have tightness on one side of the pelvis and/or sciatica.

1. Start by sitting up on your sit bones with your hands on your knees or at your hips.

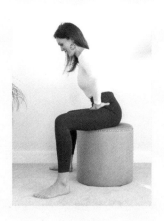

2. Lean forward from the sit bones so your bottom sticks out behind you a little. You will feel the stretch between the sit bones.

3. When you cannot move your pelvis any more, press into your heels and press your pelvis back to vertical.

Seated squat

This is similar to the hip hinge at the beginning and is a wonderful way of improving your squat by using the chair. It is great for strengthening your glutes and legs, gets the tummy working and it also trains the brain to use the hips when bending (rather than putting all the load on your lower back). Try with one leg lifted if you dare!

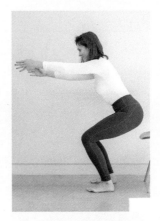

1. Start by sitting up on your sit bones with your hands on your knees. Make sure that your knees and feet are pointing forward.

2. Lean forward from the sit bones so your bottom sticks out behind you a little. You will feel the stretch between the sit bones.

3. Lift your toes and press into your heels. Keep your weight on your heels and release the toes down.

4. Breathe in, and as you keep pressing into your heels, stand up.

5. Breathe out, and as you keep pressing into your heels, sit down into the hinge.

TIP: Lifting your toes keeps the weight in your heels and makes sure that you use the backs of the legs (as the heels link up with the backs of the legs). Otherwise we can feel this in the knees. And while talking about the knees, make sure that they are tracking/facing the same direction as your toes the whole time. No knees in or out please!

Seated lunge

This is a lovely way to get the benefit of the stretchy part of a lunge as well as a little bottom muscle activation, but without it being too intense. Plus, you do not need to stand to do it, so it's easier on the balance too.

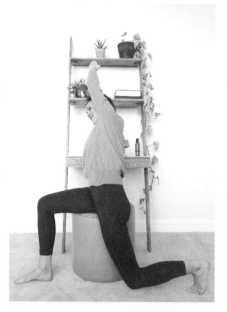

1. Sitting on your sit bones, wiggle yourself to the front of your chair. Start with your feet turned out to either side of the room, then lift your right heel and swivel yourself to the left. You will be looking left, with your left sit bone on the seat and your right sit bone off it.

2. Make sure your back heel is parallel to the front one and not turned in, as this turns your hips too. You want both hips pointing forward.

3. Press into your left heel to activate your glutes on that side.

4. Drop your right knee toward the floor to stretch the front of your thigh on this side.

5. For an extra stretch, lift your right arm up to your ear and side-bend toward the back of your chair.

6. Take a few breaths in and out here, then switch to the other side.

Hamstring stretches

There are two ways to do this movement, and I'd encourage you to try both. The first one is kinder on the hamstrings but is also good for helping you understand where your pelvis needs to be.

The hamstrings attach to behind the knee and at your sit bones, so when stretching them it's important to move from the sit bones (a la hip hinge) and not from the lower back (less effective and another extra job that the lower back does not need).

Seated hamstring stretch

1. Start up on your sit bones and wiggle your bottom to the front of your chair.

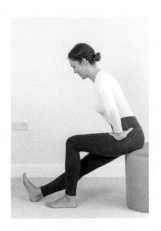

2. Take your right leg out straight, flexing your ankle and bringing your toes back toward your face. Dig your heel into the floor.

3. Breathe in and hip hinge forward while pressing into your left heel. You will feel the back of your right leg stretch.

4. Breathe out and see if you can hinge forward any more. Check that you have not shifted onto your left sit bone. Keep both pressing down.

5. Take two extra breaths in and out.

6. Move in and out of the stretch a couple of times.

7. Return to vertical and switch legs.

Standing hamstring stretch

1. Standing facing your chair, place one foot on top of the seat.

2. Check to see if your hips are level. The side of the leg you've lifted might have hitched up. Try to even the two sides out so they are horizontally level.

3. Your pelvis should be in a neutral position, so, like it was when sitting, you want your sit bones to be pointing down and not slightly forward because your bottom is tucked under.

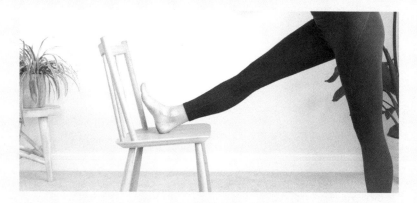

TIP: If you can't get your pelvis into a neutral position, then stick with the seated version, sitting up on your sit bones, pressing into those heels more and eventually your hamstrings will love you enough to let you move on.

4. Breathe in and hip hinge forward while pressing into your left heel. You will feel the back of your right leg stretch.

5. Breathe out and see if you can hinge forward any more. Check that you have not shifted onto your left sit bone. Keep both pressing down.

6. Take two extra breaths in and out.

7. Move in and out of the stretch a couple of times.

8. Return to vertical and switch legs.

Single leg lift seated

1. For this one you will need to shuffle to the back of your chair, but please still sit up on your sit bones.

2. Have both knees together to start.

3. Extend one leg out straight.

4. Point and flex your foot.

5. Return it to the floor and repeat on the other side.

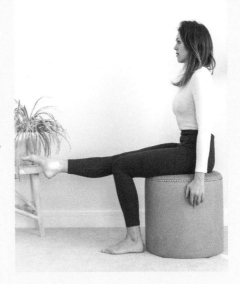

Charleston legs seated

This is a great one to do while on a video call – where no one can see your legs! – and is a nice way to get the legs moving in the hip sockets.

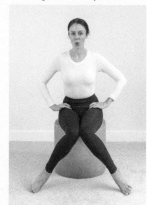

1. Sitting up on your sit bones, lift up onto the balls of both feet with your legs apart.

2. Let your knees knock against each other.

3. Let them fall out.

Standing on one leg

This is a great exercise for balance and leg, bottom and belly strength. If you struggle with balance, be sure to stand near a wall for this one!

1. Stand on your right foot and hover your left off the floor. Make sure you have your weight evenly distributed across the right foot (see page 56–7).

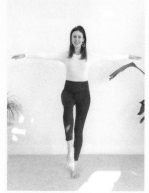

2. Lift your left leg up to a tabletop position where it is in line with the hip, creating a right angle at the knee. To challenge your balance more, lift your arms out to the side in a T shape.

3. Pop that leg down, transfer your weight to your left leg and foot and do the same on the other side.

Standing knee circles

Next up – circles! This movement is really nice for hip mobility, getting those legs to move inside the hip socket without the hip moving too (hello, pelvic stability!).

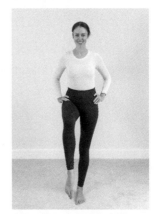

1. Lift your left leg to that tabletop position (see "standing on one leg" opposite). Make sure you have your weight evenly distributed across the right foot (as is described on page 56–7) and squeeze your right leg into the middle by engaging your inside thighs (think flamingo).

2. Check that the hips are horizontally level by pressing your left hip down and your right hip up.

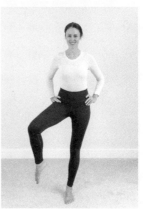

3. Place one hand on the front and the other on the back of your pelvis.

4. Imagine your leg and pelvis like a pestle and mortar. You are going to circle the pestle (leg) in the still mortar (pelvis) – hopefully without the grinding noise!

5. Make circles with your leg inside the hip socket, keeping the pelvis still.

6. Complete 3 circles in one direction, then 3 in the opposite direction and repeat with the other leg.

TIP: If you feel your pelvis moving, make the circles smaller. Once you get more stability of the pelvis and more mobility at the joint (leg moving), then increase the size of your circles.

Hip stretch

This is a lovely stretch to do standing. It feels great down the side of the body and into the front of the hip.

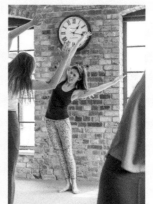

1. Stand with your heels together and your toes apart in a "V "shape.

2. Interlock your fingers and place your hands behind your head, pressing your head into your palms. Or, like I'm doing in this image, lift your arms above your head, palms facing each other for a bit of extra work.

3. Press your legs together and push your hips sideways to the left. Your spine and head will follow and go to the right.

4. Press the legs together and push your hips back to centre.

5. Repeat on the other side.

TIP: Imagine there's a tug of war between your feet and head so you are as long as possible. Imagine you are trying to lift your waist off your hips as you go up and over to each side.

Plié with heel lifts

Hello, hips! This looks akin to something you would expect to see on stage – and yes, you can look as graceful. It is an excellent movement for the entire circumference of the tops of your legs. It is strengthening and helps mobility at the hip joint.

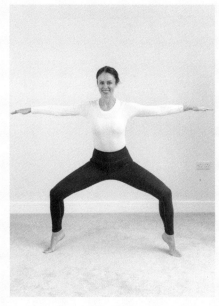

1. Stand with your legs wider than shoulder-width apart in a turned out position (so that your legs and feet are facing away from each other).

2. Do a little bend of the knees to check that the centre of your knees is aligned above your second toes. If your knees are more forward than this, then turn your feet in slightly. You could also have your arms out to the side at shoulder height, palms facing down (remember: tops of shoulders away from ears).

3. Press into your heels and the outside edge of your feet and bend your legs, trying to keep your pelvis in a vertical position.

4. Lift your heels and try to remain balanced, keeping the toes down.

5. Lower the heels and return to straight legs.

6. Repeat the bend 6–8 times, going a bit lower each time.

Leg hanging

This is an exercise I do with clients who have limited movement at the hips. With the help of gravity, these movements can lessen tightness around the hip joint in a gentle way, so they are great for anyone who feels compressed around that area. The idea is to keep the pelvis still and move the leg bone in the hip socket.

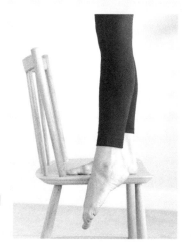

1. Stand on a raised surface so that your leg hangs without touching the floor. (I use a chair with one hand on a wall for stability – make sure you are stable and the chair is not on a wobbly surface. You can choose something lower to the ground, like a step or the stairs.)

2. Make sure you're spreading your weight evenly on the foot of your standing leg – i.e. between the heel, the ball of your big toe and the ball of the little toe.

3. Hang the other leg off the raised surface. If you squeeze your inside thighs toward each other, it will help to keep you balanced in the middle.

4. Starting small, swing your leg backward and forward. Let gravity help create space.

5. Then draw little circles with the leg in one direction and then the other.

6. Give the leg a shake.

7. Turn the leg out from the hip and then in, and give it another shake.

9. Turn around and repeat with the other leg.

The following is from my client Sarah, who suffers with osteoarthritis at the hip joint. Here, she shares with us how simple movements, such as that above, help her to move more freely and with less pain.

HOW MOVEMENT HELPS SARAH DESMOND

"My hip pain is caused by osteoarthritis, which Kerrie-Anne has helped me manage by teaching me to distinguish between my legs and pelvis. This has meant that I can walk much more easily and with less pain. I often think now in terms of lengthening my whole body and putting space into my hip joint and now feel less compressed around the top of my legs.

In practical terms this has been achieved by simple movements – moving my legs while my pelvis stays still. This is so beneficial as it eases my movement and also helps with any niggling back pain as my pelvis works more and my back feels like it does not have to work so hard and can relax!

One move I have found invaluable is 'hanging my leg'. I stand on my 'good' leg on a raised surface or step and allow the other leg to hang below, lengthening myself and creating space in my hip joint. I have been known to do this on a curb while out walking. It is such a simple and effective technique."

The roll-down

Technically this is a movement of the spine and the pelvis, but it is a nice one to add in here because it really allows you to move the two parts independently, and then feel a good stretch for your hamstrings too (while the legs stay still).

NOTE: If you are someone who has particular disc issues, osteoporosis, osteopenia or any condition where loaded flexion is contra-indicated, please do not try this one. If you are unsure then ask your medical practitioner first.

1. Begin by standing up straight.

2. Interlock your hands behind your head, press your head into your hands and keep them here until you have fully rolled down.

3. Nod your chin toward your chest (but keep pressing that head back).

4. Start to sequentially round through your back; the top of your head will go toward the floor.

5. When you cannot move your spine any more, rotate your pelvis from its vertical position to as horizontal as you can get it.

6. Drop your hands to the floor. If your fingertips do not touch, bend your legs as much as you need to.

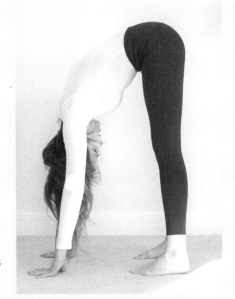

7. To roll up, rotate your pelvis back to vertical first – arms still hanging down.

8. Once your pelvis is back to vertical, roll your spine up.

NOTE: *In the image my legs are straight but the side of my hips are stacked over the side of my knee bone, which is stacked over my ankle bone. If you can roll down with straight legs, please stack your bones this way and keep your weight forward, toward the front of your feet. Try not to sink into the heels.*

Feet

Our feet do a lot of work for us, and most of us do not give them very much love at all.

In Chapter 2, I talked about improving how you stand. Specifically, I suggested spreading your weight evenly across your feet – under the heel, the ball of the big toe and the ball between the fourth and fifth toe.

Improving how you stand and move on your feet has implications for the rest of the body.

A very simple way of thinking about it is as follows:

- Your heels connect to the back of your legs and further up your body

- The outside foot connects to the outside leg and further up your body

- The inside foot (and indeed lifting your arches) connects to the inside leg and further up your body

- The front of the foot connects to the front of the body and further up your body

The more balanced we can be on our feet, the more chance we have of working in a balanced way throughout the rest of the body.

The following movements will help to make your feet stronger and more balanced, flexible and mobile, and will generally help you to move better.

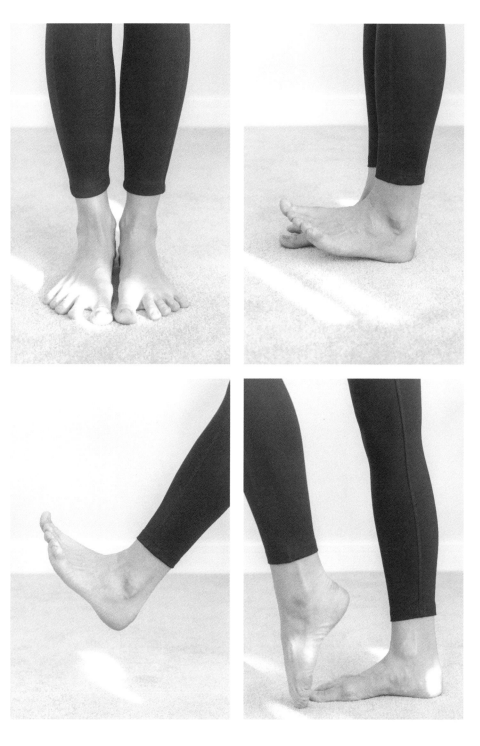

THE MOVEMENTS

These are all movements that you can do while seated. Great to do on a video call or in a meeting – assuming no one can see your feet! On page 132, I talk about foot movements you can do while standing.

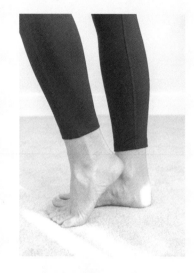

Single heel lifts

1. Seated, bring your legs together and in parallel.

2. Inhale to lift one heel.

3. Press more into the heel of the other foot.

4. Exhale to lower the heel.

5. Repeat on the other side.

Both heels

1. Bring your legs together and in parallel.

2. Inhale to lift your heels, pressing into the balls of both feet.

3. Exhale to lower your heels.

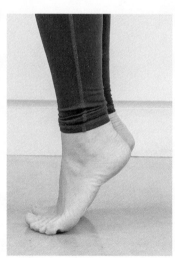

To your tip toes

1. Bring your legs together and in parallel.

2. Lift one heel to the ball of your foot.

3. Lift the ball of your foot so you are on your tip toes.

4. Return to the ball of your foot.

5. Return your heel to the floor.

6. Repeat on the other foot.

Make sure that you stay up on your sit bones for this one and you do not shift from sit bone to sit bone!

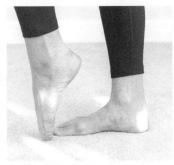

Roll your ankles

1. Bring your legs together and in parallel.

2. Lift one leg off the floor, stretching it out in front of you. Point your foot.

3. Circle your ankle a few times one way and then the other.

4. Do the same on the other foot.

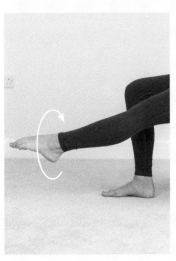

Now let's do some standing up.

Inside outside

This is fab for working the ankles but also for acquainting the two sides of each foot with the floor.

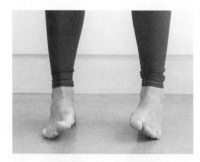

1. Stand evenly on both feet.

2. Roll onto the outside of your feet.

3. Return to centre.

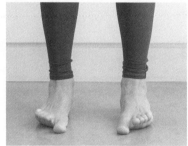

4. Roll to the inside of your feet.

5. Return to centre.

Forward and back

This is great for the ankles as well as for exploring the length of the foot.

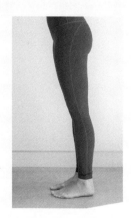

1. Stand evenly on both feet.

2. Shift your weight to the front of your foot.

3. Return to centre.

4. Shift your weight to the back of your foot.

5. Return to centre.

Spreading and lifting your toes

This is a funny exercise. I say funny because it is surprisingly difficult to do! I promise you that the more you do this one, the easier it will get – and I am speaking from first-hand "once-had-stiff-toes" experience!

Not only will this exercise help you to walk better, but it will prevent your feet from getting stiff and achy as you get older. The last step really focuses on lifting the arches of your feet, which will help with strengthening and lifting other parts of your body too, such as your inside legs and tummy muscles – woop woop! Plus, these movements also strengthen your ankles. I find they are great to do at a bus stop or when waiting for your morning coffee.

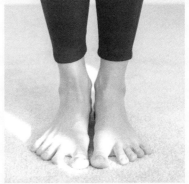

1. Start by spreading your toes really wide, trying to make as much space between each one as possible.

2. Spread them on an inhale. Relax them on an exhale. Repeat for a few breaths.

3. Spread your toes wide and inhale to lift all ten off the floor. Exhale to release them back down. Repeat a few times, trying to lift each one to the same height.

4. Leave the big toes down this time and inhale to lift the little ones up. Exhale to place them back down. Repeat for a few breaths.

5. Leave the little toes down this time and inhale to lift the big ones up. Exhale to place them back down. Repeat for a few breaths.

6. Now for the trickiest of all ... Leave the big toe and the very smallest toes down and inhale to lift the three middle ones up. Exhale to place them back down. Repeat for a few breaths.

Heel lifts

This one is good for the ankles and the backs of the legs. It also gets the inside line of your legs to work too.

1. Stand with your legs together – or as close together as is comfortable for you – and have a sense of them squeezing together like there are magnets on the inside of each leg (this will get the inside thighs to work).

2. Breathe in and lift both heels.

3. Breathe out to lower your heels.

TIP: If you squeeze your inside ankle bones, knees and thighs together, you will be more balanced doing this. Think of going straight up, rather than forward and up. And look forward (not down!).

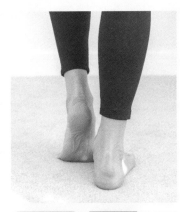

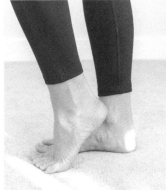

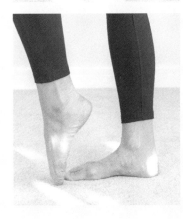

To the point

This one will work the feet as well as help you to get some hip stability work in too.

1. Stand with your legs together – or as close together as is comfortable for you – and squeeze them together like there are magnets on the inside of each leg (this will get the inside thighs to work).

2. Lift your right heel.

3. Lift up to your tip toes on the right.

4. Lower to the ball of your foot.

5. Place your heel back down.

6. Repeat on the other side.

TIP: Press your heel down on the floor to help stabilize. Make sure you focus on the bend at the front of the ankle and knee to avoid any hip hitching (keep those level). And be sure to press into the whole ball of the foot, rather than just a part, so that your heel does not go off to the left or right.

Wrists and Hands

Our hands and fingers may move to type, but it is really just a repetitive movement that we do over and over. As you now know, we want to keep our movement varied and move the body parts in all the different ways they can, so here are movements for your hands and wrists to break up the monotony of the repetitive keyboard action!

Jazz hands

If you want to be more discreet about this exercise, you can always open and close your fists while keeping your arms still in front of you (see image).

1. Bring your arms to your side and close your fists.

2. Begin to take your arms up toward your head as you open and close your fists, stretching and contracting your hands as you go.

3. Repeat the open and close as you take your hands back to your hips.

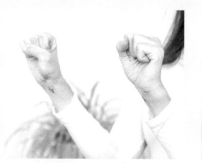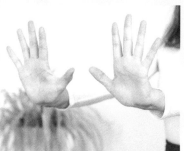

Wrist rolls

1. Make a fist with both hands.

2. Circle your wrists and hands one way.

3. Change direction and circle them the other way.

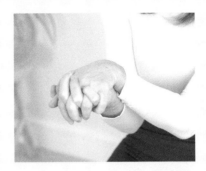

Palm stretch

1. Interlock your fingers and turn your hands so that your palms are facing away from your chest.

2. Stretch your arms forward in front of you.

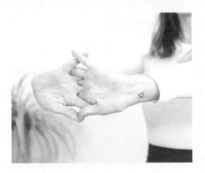

TIP: To add in some shoulder love to this one, you could take your hands above your head and back to your chest, still stretching your palms.

Karate Kid meets Vogue

1. Start with your arms down your side.

2. Take your arms out to the side and up to shoulder height (or down by your hips if this feels better).

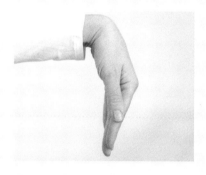 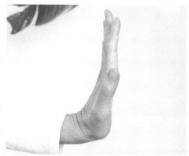

3. Turn your fingers down to the floor, bending at your wrists.

4. Turn your fingers up to the ceiling, bending the wrists the other way.

Mexican wave

1. Interlock your fingers and with floppy wrists.

2. Do a Mexican wave one way a few times and then change direction.

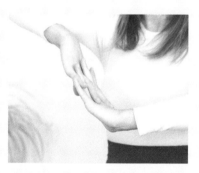

Infinity sign

1. Interlock your fingers, making a fist with both hands.

2. Draw an infinity sign with your wrists.

3. Change direction.

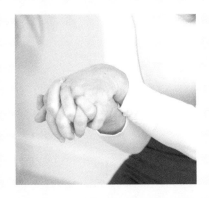

Shake them out

This is what it says on the tin – literally just shake your hands out. It's a lovely reset and a good one for getting rid of any negative tension too!

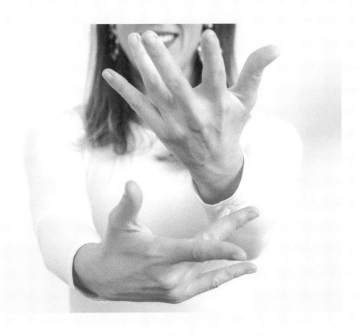

Breathing

"Are you a stingy breather? Well, don't be."

Ron Fletcher

Since it's pretty fundamental to life, breathing should be something that we can do easily and without giving it too much thought – right? If only it was that simple.

We start off well. If you watch a baby breathe, you will see the child's belly rising as they breathe in and falling as they breathe out. However, along the way, many of us lose this natural ability to do it so efficiently. Things like busyness, stress and even sucking in your tummy when you breathe in change how we breathe, and as a result we are not using our breathing apparatus to its fullest potential.

Breathe In, Breathe Out

Breathing is the exchange of gases within the body. When we breathe in, we take oxygen into the body, which we need to survive. Our lungs expand as the air comes in. Oxygen diffuses across the lungs' surface and into our bloodstreams to go to our various organs and cells. When we breathe out (exhale), our lung volume decreases and we remove extra carbon dioxide (which we do not need). We can breathe in/out through our nose or mouth.

Your diaphragm is the main muscle involved in breathing. It is a dome-shaped muscle and can be found below your lungs. When we breathe in fully, our diaphragm contracts and moves down a little, making space for the lungs to fill up and expand. At the same time, your pelvic floor (another dome-shaped muscle but this time situated in the pelvis) lengthens and descends a little to make space for the diaphragm and all the bits in between.

When you breathe out, the diaphragm relaxes and returns to its original place, and the pelvic floor (and abdominals) contract and return to their original spot.

CORE BLIMEY

Did you know that every time you take in a big breath and breathe it out, your deeper tummy muscles get involved by contracting and relaxing?

So the more you breathe big, the more your tummy is working. BONUS!

DIFFERENT TYPES OF BREATHING

There are a few different ways we can breathe. We will specifically look at four techniques here. First, the lateral (or intercostal) breath, which we will use to get movement around the ribcage and back – this is a great one for back tension. We will also look at belly breathing as a way of calming your nervous system – aka good for the mind! The next breath tries to make you as big and as wide as possible and is great for both body and mind. Lastly, the hug breath, which specifically brings focus to breathing into the back of your body but is also a lovely one to do when you feel like a little bit of nurturing (and no one else is around to do the hugging for you!).

Lateral breath

In Pilates we use a breathing technique called lateral breathing, which means breathing into the sides and back of the ribs. This is great for getting movement around the ribcage, helping to bring it into a happier position, as well as getting movement around the middle spine. It also encourages us to relax the tops of the shoulders by drawing the breath down into the bottom and sides of the lungs.

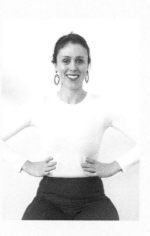

1. Place your hands on either side at the bottom of your ribs. Your thumb should be at the back and your four fingers at the front.

2. Inhale through your nose sending your breath down and out to

your hands. Your ribs will expand out to the sides. Focus especially on the back of the ribs.

3. Exhale through your mouth and your ribs will return to their start position.

4. Repeat the in- and out-breath, seeing if you can make your ribs even bigger each time.

Belly breath

I use this one when I am anxious or stressed, as it is excellent for calming the nervous system. It is also the one I would recommend if you experience tummy tension, as this type of breathing really gets the belly moving.

I start by counting to four for the inhale and four for the exhale, and then increase this to six and then maybe eight. It may help to close your eyes. Also, if you are struggling to expand your tummy on the inhale, try this one lying down on your back first, as it makes it easier. Once you've mastered that, then move to sitting.

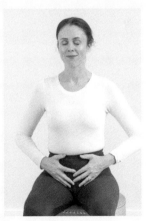

1. Place your hands on your lower tummy.

2. Inhale expanding your tummy into your hands.

3. Exhale and your tummy will draw back.

Big and wide breath

The aim is to fill your entire body with air when you inhale. While you breathe, imagine that there is a tug of war in between your sit bones and your head. Be dramatic with this one, or, as Ron Fletcher would say, "Be extravagant with your breathing and come fully alive."

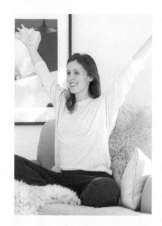

1. Put your hands by your side, palms facing out.

2. Inhale a MASSIVE breath through your nose, reaching your hands out to the side and up above your head.

3. Exhale, pressing your arms back to your side.

Hug breath

Focus your breathing into your back, as it is good for reducing tightness. I loved this one during lockdown when hugs were limited.

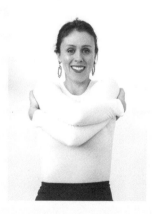

1. Give yourself a hug with your hands reaching around to your back.

2. Inhale, breathing into your back (your back will press into your hands).

3. Exhale, letting your back return to where it started.

4. Switch hands so that other is on top.

A Spotlight on Aches and Pains

"Change happens through movement, and movement heals."

Joseph Pilates

Sometimes we will experience pain in an area of the body, when the root issue is located somewhere totally different. A tight shoulder, for example, may occur because of tightness in the opposite hip, or vice versa. This has a lot to do with the connective tissue that I mentioned earlier in Chapter 1, so it's important to look at the body as a whole system, rather than just its individual parts.

When using this toolkit of movement, therefore, make sure that you mix it up. If you've got a sore shoulder, by all means roll it, but perhaps also look at what's happening at your hips. Is the opposite hip tight? If so, some leg and hip circles will help here. Perhaps the whole middle back is a bit tight? If this is the case, then you could consider taking some big ol' back breaths and then do a spot of elbow swimming.

Is your lower back hurting? Is it because you've been sat like a croissant and have been compressing your bottom spine, or perhaps you've been leaning on one side too much and the joint at the top of your pelvis is unhappy and sending lower back signals?

In order to get to the root of those aches and pains, here are some checklists you could use for some common issues. Answer each of the questions and address any that.

Lower Back Pain

This is one of the most common issues I come across, and while there is likely to be a combination of factors that give rise to your lower back pain, I would suggest focusing on each of these questions one or two at a time so you are not having to focus on too many things at once.

The checklist:

- Are you sitting up on your sit bones while working?

- Are you sitting evenly on both sit bones (i.e. not leaning more on one)?

- Are you moving your pelvis enough? Try some hip hinges (page 114) and roll downs (page 126).

- Are your ribs over your hips and not lifted up to the ceiling?

- Is your middle back tight? Try some lateral breaths (pages 142), elbow swimming (page 74) and rotation (page 93).

- Are you moving your spine enough? Try side-bends (page 91), rotation (page 93) and extension (page 97).

- Do you need to do more shake breaks (pages 67–8)?

Ache Between the Shoulder Blades

Quite often, I will be asked about aches between the shoulder blades, and while asking, the person will stretch their arms out in front of them, pulling the shoulder blades apart from each other, as though to stretch the area between them. Our brains tell us that this what we need to do, when in fact it is quite often the opposite. It is more usually the case that the area between the shoulder blades needs a bit of work, and it is the chest muscles that need the stretch (because of how we position our arms in front of us when working).

The checklist:

- Is your head hanging forward? Press your head into your hands and make sure devices are at eye height (page 84).

- Are you breathing into your middle back enough? Try lateral breathing (page 142).

- Do you need to stretch your chest? Try cactus arms (pages 76–7), hug a tree (page 78) and the door frame stretch (page 162).

- Are your shoulder blades stuck? Try polishing your halo (pages 75–6) and shoulder circles (page 73).

- Do you need to move your spine? Try side-bends (page 91), rotation (page 93) and extension (page 97).

- Do you need to be a big star and little ball more (page 101)?

Neck Pain

As discussed in the neck section, we tend to hold our head in a fixed position for long periods at a time, and for many of us this may not necessarily be a position that is great for the neck. Many of us hold tension in the tops of our shoulders and this may impact how our neck feels. Perhaps you are a jaw clencher or teeth grinder. This can also impact how your neck feels. Many people come to me with the sort of neck pain where it hurts to turn your head left and/or right, which is both unpleasant and distracting.

The checklist:

- Is your head in a good place and are your devices at eye height? Try pressing your head back into your hands more (page 84).

- Are you taking big enough breaths? Try belly breathing (page 143) and the big and wide breath (page 144).

- Do you need to roll your shoulders?

- Do you need to relax your face?

- Do you need to move your head more? Try head rotations with hands on knees (page 93–4) and the front-of-neck stretch (page 86–7).

Bottom/Hip/Pelvic Pain

The most common reason for hip pain that I come across is related to bottom-gripping (either one side or both) and holding the pelvis in a tucked-under position for long periods on a repetitive basis. One-sided bottom gripping can give you a little pelvic rotation where one side of the pelvis is more forward than the other. All this can impact the sacroiliac joint and lead to pain around the hips and bottom. Quite often I see clients for sciatica who have these things going on. The checklist below is what I would give as homework. It is also great for people who experience pain around the hip socket too.

The checklist:

- Are you sitting on both sit bones/standing evenly on both legs?

- Are you gripping your bottom and overworking some of the bottom muscles?

- Do you need to keep your pelvis stiller while moving your legs? Hello, hip stretch (page 122)!

- Do you need to work your sit bone muscles more? Do some roll downs (page 105), focusing on moving from your sit bones.

- Are your hip and leg a bit compressed? Try some standing knee circles (page 121–2) and some leg hanging (see pages 124–5), remembering to keep the pelvis still. Free up some space!

A WORD FROM
GRACE LILYWHITE

After I had my daughter Ivy, I went along to Postnatal Pilates classes with Grace Lillywhite (see page 208), an amazing Pilates teacher who specializes in women's wellness, pre- and post-natal movement and all things pelvic floor. She is a great friend of mine and a fountain of knowledge, and I wanted to share some of her wisdom here about her area of expertise:

"The way we use our bodies day to day has an important impact on our pelvic floor health. This is of utmost importance in the pre- and postnatal period because it is a time of huge transition in the bodies of women and birthing people, and we cannot underestimate the impact that this can have for the rest of their lives. 50 per cent of women over 50 experience some form of prolapse, which affects both physical and mental health. So do what you can NOW to avoid issues further down the line."

In Pregnancy

The way we sit impacts the way our pelvic floor functions, so it is important that you sit on top of your sit bones, as this will avoid the shortening and tightening of the pelvic floor that is common with our modern-day lifestyles. When the pelvic floor is over-tight, it cannot contract properly, which can impact on continence, sexual satisfaction and lower back pain. The tension you hold in your jaw can also directly reflect what is happening in your pelvis.

Women and birthing people are often told to do Kegel exercises in pregnancy, but it is really important that these are done correctly as this can also lead to a shortening and tightening of the pelvic floor if the release is not taught. The release of the pelvic floor is just as important as the contraction, so make sure you are consciously letting go of the pelvic floor after each contraction. I would also argue that (unless you have pelvic floor dysfunction and have been advised to do pelvic floor exercises by a Pelvic Health Physio) staying active and being mindful of your daily movement habits is more important.

Your posture also impacts the position of your baby and how easily your baby will move through the birth canal if you are having a vaginal birth. When you sit with your pelvis tucked under and slump backward, your baby's spine is more likely to roll toward your spine, and this can make labour a less smooth process as ideally the spine faces outward. It also restricts the amount of space your baby has to move around and get into position for birth (which is head down and spine facing outward). Creating more balance through the pregnant torso makes it easier for the baby to move through the pelvis.

Top pregnancy tips

- Sit on a Swiss ball at your desk and while watching TV if you can, as this discourages slouching and encourages movement throughout the day.

- Have an awareness of stacking your pelvis over your ankles and your ribcage over your pelvis, as this encourages good pelvic floor function and can help to reduce the severity of separation of the abdominal muscles (Diastasis Recti).

- Aim to walk 5km (3 miles) a day (unless your medical practitioner advises otherwise). You may need to build up to this slowly, but walking is amazing exercise in pregnancy and will help to keep your pelvic floor mobile and strong.

Postnatally

If you have stayed active and mobile during your pregnancy, you are more likely to have an easier postnatal recovery, but the good news is that it is never too late! Common postnatal symptoms such as pelvic floor dysfunction and abdominal separation can be addressed many years after the event, so if you are reading this with hindsight, never fear! It is a great idea to go and get a full body check by a Pelvic Health Physio or Women's Health Osteopath six to eight weeks after your baby arrives (but again, it is never too late!).

The postnatal period is usually completely exhausting and rest should always be a priority, but gently mobilizing and working on breathing patterns is essential if you want to find optimum core function.

Simple but regular things like rolling your shoulders, reaching both arms up over your head, ankle circles and going for a walk every day (when you are recovered) are great ways to start moving. Be aware of your posture when you are sitting and feeding for hours on end – again, you need to sit well to allow your body to function as you want it to.

Before you add in any high-impact exercise, **it is absolutely vital that you do a strengthening programme to support you through it.**

Top postnatal tips

- Sit on a Swiss ball, as this discourages slouching and encourages movement throughout the day (babies also like to be gently bounced in your arms on the ball, especially if you bounced on it in pregnancy).

- Address your breathing patterns. The pelvic floor moves with the breath, and making sure your breath is moving through the entire torso (especially into the bottom of the ribcage) is absolutely vital (side-bends, gentle twists and mobilizing the ribcage are all great to encourage the breath into the ribs).

- Don't rush into high-impact exercise. Build your strength first and allow your body to go into it with lots of support.

Case Study: Cathy Johnston

Job role: Lead paediatric speech and language therapist

Number of hours spent sitting for work each day: Between 7–10 hours at computer screen, with Teams meetings that are often 2 hours long.

Number of movement breaks per day: I usually feel restless on the hour, so try to move, even by just getting a drink.

Time spent moving in working day: When I work from home, I go for an early run (5–10km) to wake my body up. I do some basic PAYD stretches: side-bends, squats and split squats. When I work in the office, I cycle to and from work.

What reminds you to move? Mostly it is when I feel my energy dipping, or my eyes getting sore/fuzzy. Occasionally I can feel stiffness in my hips/ knees or hamstrings from sitting.

How does more movement make you feel? More productive – it wakes me up and reminds me to invest in my whole body. Working with Kerrie-Anne has helped me think about tiny habits and postural changes to improve my body. I now realize how stiff I had felt before doing this!

Case Study: Ian Edwards

Job role: Lawyer

Number of hours spent sitting for work each day: 10–12

Number of movement breaks per day: A lot of short breaks, but only a few minutes each. I need to take longer breaks.

How do you move during the working day? Moving by fidgeting and stretching at my desk. Working from home is not great, as being on camera means you are less likely to move around. You have to be more creative with your movement. For example, I move my legs a lot while on a video call and actively sit on my sit bones

What reminds you to move? I try to get up and move after every meeting, or every few paragraphs of a long document.

How does more movement make you feel? Really good when I consciously stretch. Sitting up on my sit bones, moving my middle back has made a big difference to how my back feels. I previously had lots of back pain and a disc issue. Since thinking about how I sit and being more conscious about moving more, my back is rarely an issue.

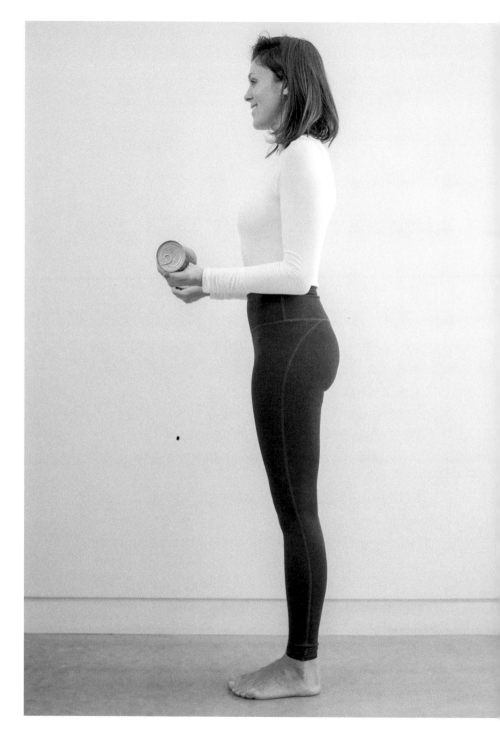

chapter 4.

Other Ways to Move While you Work

As I write this book, most of us are still working from home and may be doing so for some of the time going forward. In this chapter, I'll provide you with ideas on extra ways you can move when working from home. Assuming that a return to the office will happen in some shape or form, I have provided suggestions on how you could up your movement credit while at the office too.

GET YOUR TINS OUT!

Not all of us have weights at home (or even want to have weights at home!), but I am guessing most of us have tinned food in the cupboard. You can use your tins of beans (chickpeas, tomato soup, whatever ... !) to add weight to the following movements, though they all work well without them too, if you prefer. Arm and shoulder work, here we come!

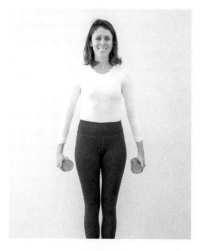
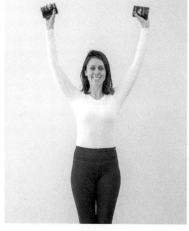

Arms up and down

1. Start by holding your arms down by your side, palms facing out with your tins in your hands.

2. Breathe in and lift your arms up above your head. Drop the tops of your shoulders down and away from your ears as your arms go above your head.

3. Breathe out to return your arms to your hips.

Elbows in, forearms out

This is a great exercise for working the back of the shoulders, stretching the chest and strengthening the arms.

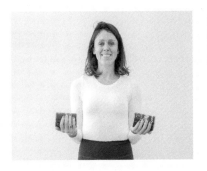 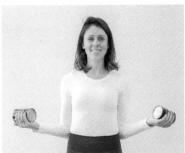

1. Start by holding your arms in at your side, elbows at a right angle so your forearms are pointing forward, palms facing up to the ceiling with your tins in your hands.

2. Take your forearms away from each other and out to the side (elbows stay in).

3. Bring them back.

Arm circles

1. Holding your tins, reach your arms down to the floor and press the tops of your shoulders away from your ears.

2. Squeeze the back of your armpits as you lift your arms out to the side and up to shoulder height, palms down.

3. Drop the tops of your shoulders even further away from your ears.

4. Start to draw little circles with your arms, a few times in one direction and then in the other.

TIP: Press into the tins with your little fingers to help activate the back of the armpit muscles. Relax your thumb press a little, as these link up to the tops of the shoulders and we don't want those guys taking over.

Shoulder press

1. With the tins in your hands, bend your elbows, have your hands in line with the front of your shoulders and your palms facing forward.

2. Reach your arms up above your head (remember: tops of shoulders away from your ears) until your arms are straight.

3. Return your arms to chest height.

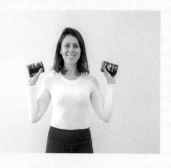
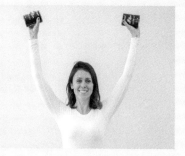

USING YOUR HOME AS YOUR EQUIPMENT

A great thing you could do is to take advantage of the props that are permanent fixtures in your home. Here are a few suggestions:

Kitchen bench stretch

This is a favourite of my good friend and first mentor, Sarah Woodhouse.

1. Place your hands on your kitchen bench, sink, etc.

2. Walk your feet back until your back is the same level as your hands. You want a flat back while honouring the natural curves of the spine, so you may need to bend your knees and stick your bottom out.

3. Imagine you are pulling the kitchen counter apart while at the same time pushing it away. Keep your head between your arms.

4. Breathe in and, when you breathe out, lift your ribs to increase the stretch (sort of in the armpit area).

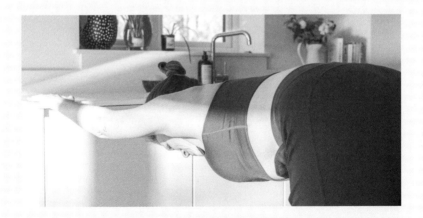

Door frame stretch

This is very simple but great for stretching your chest.

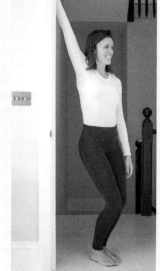

1. Place your right arm straight (but not with a locked elbow!) up one side of a door frame, palm facing the frame.

2. Turn the rest of your body away from the arm and bend your legs a little.

3. Come back to centre and repeat a couple of times before moving on to the other side.

Sofa back extension

Ah, the ad break! This exercise is a favourite of mine. I sit toward the back of the sofa, up on my sit bones, hands behind my head, and extend my spine over the back of the sofa.

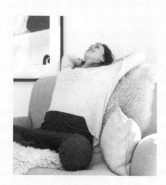

If you don't have a sofa that enables this, then try to remember to move every so often when watching TV and frequently change the position you are in while watching.

Ironing board standing desk

I remember doing at interview for the *Sunday Times Style* magazine and was told that one of the journalists was using an ironing board as a standing desk. I thought this was a genius idea. You can alter the height to suit you too!

Anyone for tennis?

A tennis ball can be great for working your feet, because it can help with "unbunching" that fascia at the bottom of the foot. It can also help you get closer to being able to touch your toes. Once you've done the first foot and placed it down, I guarantee it will feel so much more spread out than the other one.

1. Roll the ball under one foot, moving it from front and back.

2. Draw circles with it under your arches.

3. Try to pick the ball up with your toes.

4. Switch to the other foot.

TIP: Try keeping a tennis ball under your desk, then you can introduce this movement alongside other work tasks – for example, when in a Zoom meeting.

ROLL WITH IT!:
THREE THINGS TO DO WITH TENNIS BALLS (THAT AREN'T TENNIS!)

Tessa Clist (see page 208) is a Pilates teacher who originally trained as a massage therapist. She's a big fan of using the tennis ball and so I asked her to share some of her top tips and techniques:

"I love showing people how to use simple self-massage techniques to help ease tired and aching knotty muscles. Balls are my friends, and I have them in all different sizes and textures. A tennis ball is a great thing to use for self-massage and is easily obtainable. Here are three of my clients' favourite simple techniques that can be done with tennis balls to wake up tired feet, ease sore, crunchy shoulders and help with cranky knees."

These techniques are perhaps no replacement for a good, proper massage, but they are a great thing to do between sessions – and they're free! Some words of advice before you embark on your self-massage:

- GO EASY: If a certain spot hurts, then back off! If it feels the right side of sore, then carry on, but do so with care. We have become used to thinking that harder is better with massage, but on the contrary: soft tissue responds wonderfully well to a gentler touch.

- GO SLOWLY: Soft tissue (the muscles and the fascia that wraps around and betwixt all our muscles) responds to S-L-O-W movement. The slower the better!

- SHORT AND SWEET: You might think that the more the better here, but actually two or three minutes on each area is the most beneficial amount of time to spend.

- RELAX AND BREATHE: These techniques are more effective if you relax and breathe while you do them! Take a moment to stop, breathe and let yourself melt onto the ball.

Foot refresh

You can do this seated or standing, but preferably barefoot. Bear in mind that it will feel stronger if you stand.

1. Take a moment to focus on how your feet both feel. Move them around, give your toes a wiggle, look at the colour of them.

2. Start by placing the ball under the centre of your heel. Ease your weight slowly onto the ball then off a few times.

3. Roll the ball up a little so that it is just before the centre/arch of the foot. From here you can ease on and off the ball again, then roll the foot from side to side over the ball.

4. Next move to the centre of the foot. This is usually the most tender area of the foot, so go gently! Here, you can start kneading the ball in small circles with your foot.

5. Next, place the ball of your foot on the ball and rest the heel on the floor (in standing, this gives your Achilles' tendon and lower calf a nice stretch). Then slowly, but as firmly as you can manage, roll the ball from toes to heel, then lightly back to the toes again. Repeat this a few times.

6. Finish off by rolling the ball all around the sole of your foot, honing in on any areas that feel like they need it.

7. When you step off the ball, see if you feel the difference. You might even notice that the colour of your foot may have changed!

8. Repeat on the other foot.

Knee de-crankifier

This is great for those with slightly cranky knees. You need two tennis balls and a sock for this. Pop the tennis balls inside the sock and knot the end so that the balls are sitting snugly next to each other.

1. Start by lying on the floor on your side, propping yourself up on your elbow if you wish.

2. Place the socked-balls beneath the leg that's on the floor, near but not right on the knee, so that the leg rests between the two balls.

3. Let your leg be heavy and relaxed on the balls, then VERY SLOWLY start to bend and straighten the underneath leg.

4. You can vary the position on the leg. Moving the balls up a little can be tender, so go easy, and if it doesn't feel right then stop!

5. Repeat on the other side.

Shoulder easer

You will need one ball and a patch of wall or a sturdy door for this one.

1. In standing, take a moment to assess how your shoulders are feeling. Does one feel higher, tighter or achier than the other? If you roll them around, do they sound crunchy or clicky?

2. Use your hands to feel for the overworked, tight muscles at the top of the shoulders (trapezius). This is where we will nestle the ball.

3. Then lean against the wall with the ball between you and get rolling!

4. Focus on the muscle and fleshy areas rather than bone and apply as much pressure as you feel OK with, rolling slowly around the muscle, just as if a masseuse has their thumbs in just the right spot!

5. Try locating the ball between your shoulder blade and spine on that side. Pinning the ball in place with your body, you can move up and down slowly, and try lifting your arm up and down slowly.

6. Roll your shoulders around, and compare how this shoulder now feels to the other shoulder.

7. Then repeat on the other side.

You will look kind of weird doing this exercise, so you might want to warn any colleagues if you are doing this at work! Even better, get them to try it after you – their shoulders will thank you!

Dance, Dance, Dance!

I think everyone should do more dancing. I highly recommend simply whacking on your favourite tune and moving to it. As Martha Graham once said: "Nobody cares if you dance well. Just get up and dance."

Kids are great dancing buddies, and it give the whole exercise more silliness, fun and purpose. But seriously, even if you just manage a two-step while you're stirring your pasta this evening, I guarantee you will feel happier for it. If you like listening to music while you work, you could even have a little bop as you type!

As Jenna Zaffino (see page 208), movement expert and educator, says:

"Let your sit sessions be their own fun event. Choose a great playlist and wiggle around while you work. It will pass the time and lift your spirits."

Bounce, Bounce, Bounce!

I am a big fan of the rebounder – a mini trampoline. It is so hard to be angry when you bounce, and you can put it somewhere like the kitchen (which is where mine is) so that every time you are waiting for the kettle to boil or for dinner to cook, you can have a little jump.

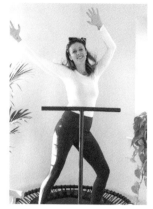

You could put it near your workspace and jump whenever you are in "thinking" mode (which is exactly what I have been doing while writing this book). You could also do what Pilates instructor Anya Hayes (@mothers.wellness.toolkit) does and set a timer on your phone on the hour every hour and get up and bounce for five minutes to get your heart rate going and energize your brain. Every little helps!

Walk Outside

Obviously, this is not one that happens at our desk, but it really is one of my favourite ways to move during the day from both a physical and mental perspective. Even just 10 or 20 minutes of walking outside is beneficial. Ask yourself this: have I ever felt worse for getting out for a walk? I suspect the answer is no.

Extra Ways to Move at Work

When at the office, we can up our incidental movement by attaching extra movement to tasks we are doing. The following suggestions will not be an option for everyone, of course, but try to incorporate some/all of these into your day:

*Note: **These should not replace our Move More Moves; think of them as a supplement to the amount we are moving!***

- Take the stairs wherever possible. This includes in tube/train stations too. Walk up the escalator too, where you can.

- Get off public transport earlier/park your car further away to walk. Better still is to walk or cycle to work if that is an option.

- Schedule walking meetings if possible. This is a great one to do when you do not have lots of papers, etc.

- Go to the bathroom/bin/printer that is furthest away from your desk.

- Go and physically speak to colleagues at their desk rather than email where you can.

- Have a glass of water on your desk rather than a bottle so you need to make regular trips to the kitchen.

- Go out for a walk at lunchtime.

- Walk whenever you take a call.

Case Study: Lydia Woods

Job role: Executive Assistant

Number of hours spent sitting for work each day: 8–10

Number of movement breaks per day: I try to move at least once every 1–2 hours. Since doing PAYD, I also do a lot of movement while seated too. The beauty of that being that you do not have to leave the seat to actually move.

Time spent moving in working day: When commuting, a typical day is: 30 mins walk in the morning/30 mins walk at lunch/30 mins at the end of the day. When working from home, I get out every day for 5–6km (3–4 miles). I also do a lot of incidental movement while seated, getting up to get water/lunch, etc.

How do you move when at your desk? I follow the PAYD day-to-day moves – they are easy and have become a habit.

What reminds you to move? I consciously make an effort to stand up/move, ensuring I take screen breaks.

How does more movement make you feel? Refreshed, happy and motivated.

Case Study: Claire Edwards

Job role: Lawyer

Number of hours spent sitting for work each day: 9

Number of movement breaks per day: 2 plus lunch – usually stretching when making tea or during calls, etc.

Time spent moving in working day: 1–2 hours

How do you move when at your desk? I do the moves I learned when Kerrie-Anne gave a class at my law firm. For example, shoulder circles; lifting my legs and flexing; putting my hands behind my head and lifting backward over my chair; bouncing on my sit bones! On long calls, I stand up and stretch from side to side; I go up and down onto tip toes; I stretch my legs. Thankfully my calls aren't video calls!

What reminds you to move? I now find it natural to do a few movements every now and then. I sit more on my sit bones – imagining Kerrie-Anne telling me to!

How does more movement make you feel? The movements, while simple, make a massive difference to my mobility and comfort.

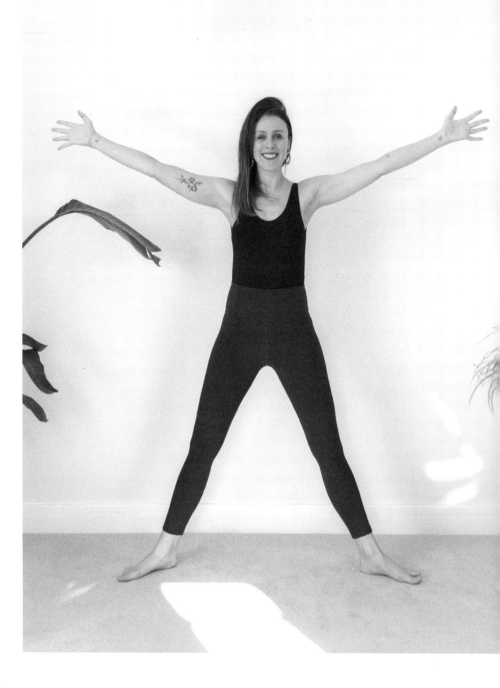

chapter 5.

Setting Yourself Up For More Movement

It is all very well knowing the movements, but the most challenging part for most of us is figuring out, and remembering, when to do more movement. It's easy to get into work mode and then struggle to get out of it when we are super focused. This section is intended to give you some ideas on how you could go about incorporating more movement into your day, while recapping on some points we introduced earlier.

Change How You Speak About Movement

Ditch the word "exercise" if it makes you automatically think you do not have enough time to do it and talk about "moving your body" instead. I call it getting in your "move more moves", but you can make up your own word for it if that helps. It does not really matter, as long as it gets you moving more. Whatever language you use, aim to frame it as more of a joy and less of a chore!

Keep it Simple

The moves in this book are intended to be accessible. You should be able to do them in whatever clothes you are wearing (i.e. so that you do not need to bring a change of clothes, and then take time changing clothes to do the moves). It is also the case that you do not need a large or dedicated space to do them. Keeping it simple means you are more likely to do it, and it saves on time too.

Change How You Think About Sitting

We need to change our mindset when it comes to sitting and recognize that sitting still for long, uninterrupted periods at a time every day is damaging to our health. We need to find ways of mitigating the impact of lots of sitting by sitting in active ways, standing more and embracing movement as much as we can. Much in the same way as eating more vegetables is good for us, credit in the movement bank is what it is all about. BE A FIDGET!

Do Stuff That Makes You Smile

"We don't stop playing because we grow old; we grow old because we stop playing."

George Bernard Shaw

For me, this is what it is all about. If we enjoy the movement we do, we are more likely to do it. Shake breaks, engaging in a spot of bottom shuffling, being a big star and a little ball, dancing, bouncing, walking out in nature, playing "tag "or "guess the animal through actions" with your children are all ways you could move that bring a smile to your face.

Check in on How Movement Makes You Feel

This is closely linked to doing stuff that makes you smile. Every time you move, take a moment at the end to think about how you feel. You are more likely to do something that makes you feel good, so once you have registered that feeling, you will be more likely to move more going forward.

Move While You Wait

An excellent time to move is while you are waiting for something to happen, and there will be many opportunities for this during your day. For example, when you brush your teeth in the morning. Assuming you brush your teeth for two minutes, you could stand on one leg to do leg circles for a minute and then switch over to the other leg. (Just try not to get the toothpaste on your face!)

Here are some other suggestions for moving while you wait:

- Lift your heels while you dry your hair

- Stretch in the kitchen while you wait for the kettle to boil

- Big breaths while the shower heats up

- Take shake breaks while waiting for meetings to start

- Toe lifts while waiting in a queue

- Shake it out while the adverts or recaps run on the TV

- Wrist rolls while your computer loads

Attach Movement to Things You Already Do

As well as moving while you wait for everyday things to happen, by linking a particular movement to an existing everyday task, the task becomes the "reminder" to move. For example:

- When you turn your computer on in the morning, sit on your sit bones for the first five minutes

- When you switch on the computer in the morning, take five big breaths

- Raise and lower your heels six times when you press "go" on the coffee machine

- Stand up and wiggle every time you get a glass of water (water is a fantastic movement enabler)

- Move your spine at the end of every meeting

- Walk to get your lunch (preferably outside)
- Every time you speak on the phone, draw circles with your nose to mobilize your neck

I suggest that you write down three of your own movement enablers and stick them somewhere visible. The more specific they are, the more likely you are to do it, and the more likely it will be to become an additional incidental movement you do.

HOW MOVEMENT HELPS

Here's how Tannis Bridge, a holistic therapist who specializes in massage, introduces additional movement into her day:

"If I am resisting committing to my morning routine, I like to sneak some squats, stretches and lunges into my everyday movement. I will lift my heels while doing the washing up, stretch my hamstrings while brushing my teeth, squat while I empty the dishwasher and side stretch while the kettle boils.

If you make it a habit, it all adds up, and it is fun to think up new ways to enhance the daily chores. I also like to stand on one leg at every opportunity (giving both a go, of course) to work on my balance."

Have Visual Reminders

Visual cues are a great way of reminding yourself to move – even something as simple as a good old Post-it note at your desk will do. The screen saver on your phone or laptop is another good place to have a visual reminder (sorry, kids, partners and pets!).

Set Alarms

You could try setting an alarm that reminds you to move on your phone or computer. You may even have one of those snazzy watches that reminds you to move. If you are someone who presses snooze when the alarm goes off, then put the reminders on a device that you can put out of arm's reach, so at the very least you have to get up to turn off the alarm!

Buddy Up With Someone

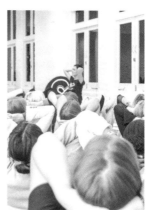

Schedule meetings into your calendar where you move with another person. It could be that you put together a short routine based on the exercises in this book and then you do them together, say for five minutes a few times a week. This way you hold each other accountable too.

The other benefit of buddying up with others is that you can start to copy each other (and hopefully the good bits!). I notice this all the time when socializing with friends. More often than not, someone will comment on my posture and say things like, "You are making me want to sit up straight," and soon everyone will start to sit up differently.

Take Back-To-Back Meeting Movement Breaks

Whether you are working from home or at the office, back-to-back meetings leave little room for movement (although there's arguably more where you are in the office and have to move from room to room). Here are some ideas to introduce movement on days filled with meetings:

- Where you can, schedule a walking meeting. Ideally it would be those where you do not need papers and can easily walk and talk (in the home-working scenario, this would be a "video-off" meeting).

- Move before the meeting starts, either by walking around the room or wiggling your legs under the table (if working from home, turn your video off while waiting for all participants to join the meeting).

TIP: Talk to your colleagues about movement breaks in meetings. I worked with a group of NHS nurses who decided that at they would start each team meeting with a few minutes moving around.

Another team in Bournemouth decided to have a team movement break every day at 11am (they moved along to my Instagram videos, picking a different one each day).

Follow Along to Someone You Love on Social Media

There are so many movement teachers out there sharing tips, videos and inspiration. So why not choose someone you love and check in on them once a day? (You could even follow me if you fancy @pilatesatyourdesk!) You could even turn a notification on so you are prompted whenever they share something – a prod from afar, shall we say! Studies show that moving along with someone is not only a great way to hold you accountable but it is also good for your self-esteem.

Sign Up to Move With Me

I offer workshops to businesses online around the world and in person around the UK. I also have a subscription service for businesses offering a bank of videos of varying length for you to do whenever you like, as well as several short live sessions per week. You could do the videos at home, in the office or wherever. You can find out more about that on my website: www.pilatesatyourdesk.com.

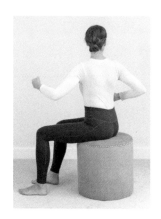

Try to Structure Movement Into Your Day

Like with many other aspects of our lives, when it comes to movement, having some sort of routine will help you to make sure that you move. Now, I appreciate that the same things are unlikely to happen every day, especially where your work diary moves around a lot, etc, so it may be difficult to make a plan to schedule in movement.

Given this, it could be an idea to think of your day more generally, and this is what I suggest in my Pilates At Your Desk workshops. The following plan is intended to help you structure more movement into your day when working from home:

1. As soon as you open your eyes each morning, take some big breaths. Set a number based on what is realistic for you – even one deep breath is better than none! It sets the tune for the day, wakes up your body, gives you a stretch and you do not even have to move!

2. Do some movement before you start work. Whether this be a 20-minute session of something you love, or adding in movement to your routine by moving while you wait (see pages 190–5).

3. As soon as you turn on your computer, sit on your sit bones. Even if just for five minutes each day. Over time you will create a new habit and build on core strength. Eventually, you'll be able to sit this way for longer.

4. Schedule movement breaks into your diary. Every 20–30 minutes is the ideal, but do what is manageable for you. Just a minute or two each time. **If you're someone who will ignore the reminder, put the reminders on a device you can have on the other side of the room. Then, at the very least, you'll get up to switch off the alarm.** You can use your PAYD toolkit of movements for inspiration on ways to move. Keep it varied!

5. Have a celebratory movement session at the end of the working day. This will serve as a positive boundary between work and leisure time. You could be a big star and little ball, or have a shake out, or even put on your favourite tune for a kitchen boogie!

Keep it Manageable

"Don't try to rush progress. Remember – a step forward, no matter how small, is a step in the right direction. Keep believing."

Kara Goucher

A WORD FROM
EMMA BRAY

Here are some more wise words from my friend, Emma Bray (see page 208). Emma is a Pilates educator who teaches Pilates, yoga and HIIT, and here is what she had to say about choosing the right moves for you:

"Figure out what works best for you. We are all different. What one person enjoys will be another's worst nightmare! I'm easily bored with cardio, so I mix it up with HIIT, dancing, walking quickly up hills or the stairs, skipping, gymnastics ribbons (honestly, I have two in my front room!) and strength training. I like using my own body weight and I live in a small space, so HIIT, Pilates, yoga, free weights, lifting shopping bags (I'll do a few bicep curls with mine) are movements I can do at home, or if I'm feeling sociable/have time, I'll join a class.

Become curious and inventive with your movement or copy another's until you find what works for you."

This is key. If you decide that every time you send an email you are going to run for 30 minutes, then (unless you are someone who sends very few emails and loves running) you are probably setting yourself up for failure.

If, on the other hand, you say that every time you finish two paragraphs in a document you will pick a move from this book, doing a different one each time, then that is more likely to be something that you can commit to.

Making It Culturally Acceptable to Move Within Your Workplace

I asked a client what would make her move more during the working day and she said, "If it was culturally acceptable to take movement breaks within the working day." This is interesting, particularly when you review the "cultural acceptance" of employees taking multiple cigarette breaks. At an office where I used to work, people would get up and leave every hour for a 10-minute cigarette break. Can you imagine if we felt empowered to do that for a "walking break"?

I've worked with lots of businesses over the past few years where movement is actively encouraged, as they know the benefits this brings to working life, wellbeing and productivity as a whole, and that's why they bring me in to show employees how and when to do it.

If everyone is moving at work, then movement becomes normal. If no one is moving, then yes, you may feel a bit odd in the corner doing your stretches, or have to surreptitiously take it into the loos and then have your colleagues wonder why you go to the loo every hour for 5 minutes! So, let's normalize what our bodies are made to do.

Case Study: Emma-Victoria Farr

Job role: Financial journalist

Number of hours spent sitting for work each day: 9

Number of movement breaks per day: 2–3

Time spent moving in working day: 1 hour

How do you move when at your desk? Short PAYD breaks by following along to Kerrie-Anne on Instagram, joining one of her classes on the PAYD platform, or a walk around the house/garden/beyond. Moving with PAYD always makes me smile, and I've even got my mother onboard!

What reminds you to move? When I feel my muscles stiffening up with stress, or I think of Kerrie-Anne!

How does more movement make you feel? Amazing. Immediately all the tension building up dissipates and I feel less stressed.

Case Study: Amy

Job role: Events Co-ordinator

Number of hours spent sitting for work each day: 6–7

Number of movement breaks per day: Around 5–6 breaks to stand up and move around, and then I move a lot at my desk thanks to Pilates At Your Desk!

Time spent moving in working day: 2–3 hours

How do you move when at your desk? I tend to do some stretches, mostly arm stretches, and make sure I'm sitting on my sit bones! I've recently got some wireless headphones, so I can stand up and walk around while on virtual meetings/calls.

What reminds you to move? Seeing prompts from PAYD Instagram stories! The need for a cup of tea, and using a glass for water so I need to get up regularly to fill it.

How does more movement make you feel? It makes me feel better; I feel more focused and energized.

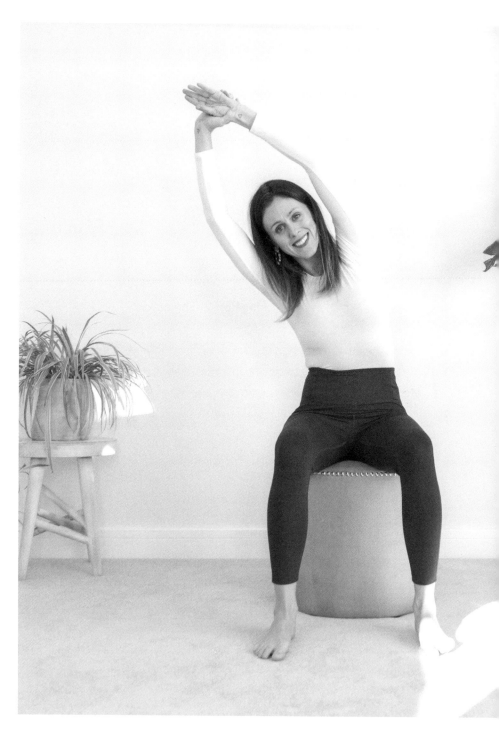

chapter 6.

Some Suggested Mini Movement Routines

Here are some combinations that you could do. Each combination of six moves allows you to try to keep them short and varied. You can do these routines as they are, or use them as a base and put your own together. Remember: if in doubt, shake it out! I would do six to eight repetitions of each movement. When you are moving each side separately, do 3–4 repetitions on each side.

A Morning Routine

This is a great routine that you can do seated on the side of your bed.

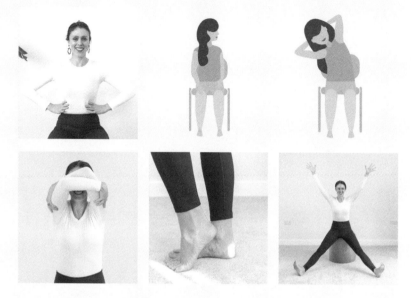

- Lateral breath (pages 142–3)

- Rotation with hands on knees (pages 93–4)

- Side-bend (page 91)

- The mighty yawn (page 80)

- Heel lifts (page 134)

- Big star (page 101)

Routines for Between Meetings

Here are two quick routines you could do before meetings:

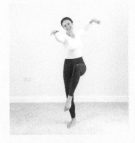
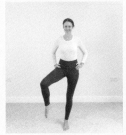
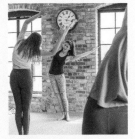
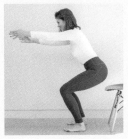
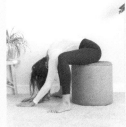
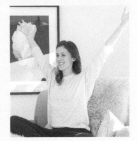

1. First routine

- Shake break (pages 67–8)

- Standing knee circles (page 121)

- Hip stretch (page 122)

- Seated squat (pages 114–5)

- Back flop (page 100)

- Big and wide breath (page 144)

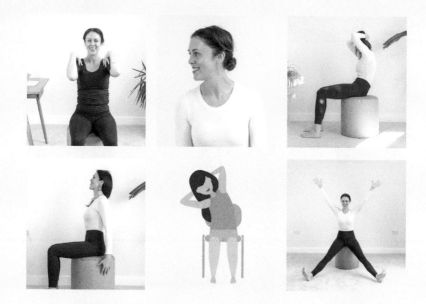

2. Second routine

- Elbow circles (page 74)

- Neck rotation (page 93)

- Flex your spine from bottom to top (page 96)

- Extend the upper spine (page 97)

- Side-bend (page 91)

- Rotation with legs and arms in a "V" (pages 94–5)

Beat the Afternoon Slump

This routine will energise you and is also a great one to do when having a creative/productive lull.

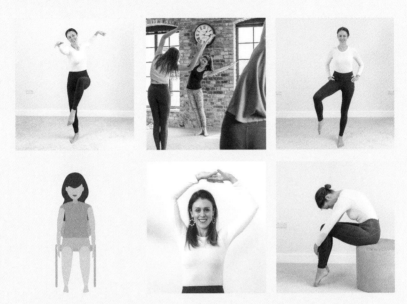

These can be done standing:

- Shake break (pages 67–8)

- Hip stretch (page 122)

- Standing knee circles (page 121)

The rest can be done seated:

- Shoulder circles (page 73–4)

- Polishing the top of your halo (pages 75–6)

- Star and ball (page 101)

Neck & Shoulder Tension

Big breaths are your best friend when it comes to these areas so this is where we will begin.

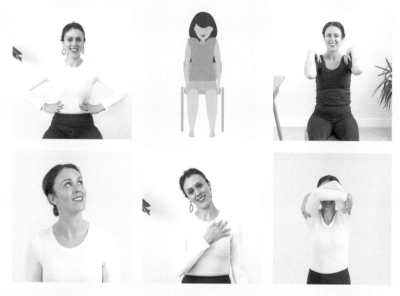

- Lateral breath (pages 142–3)

- Lift and melt (page 73)

- Elbow circles (page 74)

- Head circles with eyes (pages 85–6)

- Front-of-neck stretch (pages 86–7)

- The mighty yawn (page 80)

Discreet Desk Session

Moves that you can do while seated in front of your screen – in the office – with your headset on.

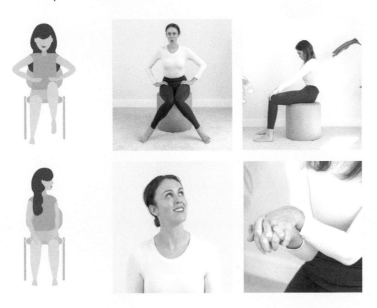

- The march (page 112)

- Charleston legs seated (page 120)

- Cat/cow, with hands on knees (page 98)

- Rotation with hands on knees (pages 93–4)

- Head circles with eyes (pages 85–6)

- Wrist rolls (page 137)

Case Study: Rachael Savage

Job role: Chartered accountant

Number of hours spent sitting for work each day: 7

Number of movement breaks per day: Daily exercise, plus a couple of movement breaks each day.

Time spent moving in working day: A couple 10-minute movement breaks, plus 45–60 minutes of exercise.

How do you move when at your desk? I do a 10-minute stretch morning and evening, usually cat/cow, child's pose, as well as spine rotations at my chair. I'm always jiggling my legs up and down under my desk to give movement!

What reminds you to move? I've scheduled reminders into my diary! Mid-morning, when I think it's time to put the coffee machine on, I do 10 minutes of movement first and then mid-afternoon, when I hear the school buses pull into the car park, it's time to do the same!

How does more movement make you feel? It clears my head and helps me feel less stiff.

Case Study: Gillian Davison

Job role: Talent Acquisition Manager

Number of hours spent sitting for work each day: 8

Number of movement breaks per day: 3

Time spent moving in working day: 1 hour

How do you move when at your desk? Simple stretches while sitting, with neck rolls being a particular favourite. I'm also really mindful of sitting up on my sit bones.

What reminds you to move? I create diary reminders and treat my micro movement breaks like any other meeting!

How does more movement make you feel? By moving more, I feel energized and my work productivity increases. It also boosts my mental wellbeing.

Et Voilà!

I hope you have enjoyed moving with me and will keep this book on your desk as a visual reminder to move. Remember, the best you can do for your body is to move it often and keep the movement varied. Yes, go along to that gym or dance class you love, but also integrate more movement into your day. Let movement deficits be a thing of the past – it is time to keep our movement bank in credit! I promise you will feel better for it.

Thank you for taking the time to move with me.

Kerrie-Anne

About the Author

Kerrie-Anne Bradley is a self-professed ex-professional sloucher, Pilates teacher and founder of Pilates At Your Desk, a programme of simple movements you can do while working at your desk.

She is passionate about movement, splitting her time between working with individuals, groups and businesses. She works with those with ongoing conditions such as arthritis, osteoporosis, sciatica, spinal injuries and many other conditions, as well as with international businesses, from global tech companies to international banks and law firms. Her workshops 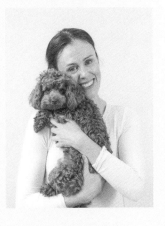 not only help people to sit, stand and move better while they work, but they are also great for producitvity, mental health and team building.

Kerrie-Anne believes in bringing joy to movement. She loves a little boogie and can be found to deliver movement with a gigantic smile. She is so eager to get as many people moving as possible that she recently launched an online platform called "move at your desk" where you can find videos and live movement sessions each week.

Find out more: @pilatesatyourdesk | www.pilatesatyourdesk.com

Acknowledgements

Thank you to everyone at Watkins for your support in bringing this book to life, especially to Anya for commissioning me and to Brittany for being an editing whizz. Thank you also to all of the amazing photographers, Chloe Williams, Stacey Horler, Amy Whittingham, Charlotte Green, Josh Tucker and Will Pyne and the illustrator, Johanna Arajuuri, who brought my movements to life.

Thank you to everyone who has contibuted to this book. I want to say a special thank you to Emma Bray, Grace Lillywhite, Grace Hurry, Jenna Zaffino, Julie Driver, Kath Pentecost, Sarah Woodhouse and Tessa Clist – all of whom I have been lucky to learn from over the years.

I would like to add an extra special mention to Sarah Woodhouse. Without you I wouldn't be the teacher I am today and I'm incredibly grateful for all the support, knowledge and wise words you shared with me in those early days.

Thank you also to Professor Fehmidah Munir for contributing your research and knowledge to this book. And to Dr Katharine Ayivor-Nygard for sharing your thoughts. Thank you also to my wonderful clients for being case studies.

Thank you to my husband Tim and the friends who read this book. And lastly a mention to my daugter Ivy who has the best moves of anyone I know: you are a superstar and I love you very much.

Notes

1   Casperan et al., 1985

2   www.who.int/news/item/25-11-2020-every-move-counts-towards-better-health-says-who

3   Benatti, 2015

4   Dempsey et al., 2016, 2018

5   Loh et al., 2020

6   Mackie et al., 2019

7   Buckley et al., 2015

8   Straker et al., 2013

9   The new WHO guidelines on physical activity and sedentary behaviours were published on 26 November 2020. The launch webinar introduced participants to the new WHO Guidelines on physical activity and sedentary behaviour and five panellists from around the world discussed the importance of guidelines for their work and the promotion of physical activity for physical activity for everyone, everywhere. www.who.int/news-room/events/detail/2020/11/26/default-calendar/webinar-who-2020-guidelines-on-physical-activity-and-sedentary-behaviour

10   Kandola et al., 2020

11   drchatterjee.com/bitesize-how-10-minutes-of-exercise-a-day-
        can-improve-mental-health-dr-brendon-stubbs/

12   My friend Nichola Joss (@nicholajoss on Instagram) has some
        lovely facial massage videos that you can follow. She did lots
        of these throughout lockdown and I found these made a
        massive different to how my very tight jaw felt.

13   Pez comes from the sweets container that has a shuttle of
        sweets with a head on top. It moves up and down while the
        sweets shoot out of the mouth.

Bibliography

Benatti FB, Ried-Larsen M. (2015) "The effects of breaking up prolonged sitting time: a review of experimental studies." Med Sci Sports Exerc 47(10): 2053–2061.

Buckley JP, Hedge A, Yates T, Copeland RJ, Loosemore M, Hamer M, Bradley G, Dunstan DW. (2015) "The sedentary office: an expert statement on the growing case for change toward better health and productivity." Br J Sports Med 49(21): 1357–62. doi: 10.1136/bjsports-2015-094618.

Casperan CJ, Powell KE, Christenson, GM. (1985) "Physical activity, exercise, and physical fitness: definitions and distinctions for health-related research." Public Health Rep 100(2): 126–131. www.ncbi.nlm.nih.gov/pmc/articles/PMC1424733/

Chatterjee, R. (12 February 2020) Podcast: "How Exercise Changes Your Brain and Reduces Your Risk of Depression with Brendon Stubbs." drchatterjee.com/how-exercise-changes-your-brain-and-reduces-your-risk-of-depression/

Dempsey, PC, Larsen, RN, Winkler, EAH, Owen, N, Kingwell, BA, Dunstan, DW. (2018) "Prolonged uninterrupted sitting elevates postprandial hyperglycaemia proportional to degree of insulin resistance." Diabetes, Obesity and Metabolism 20(6): 1526–30. doi.org/10.1111/dom.13254

Dempsey, PC, Sacre, JW, Larsen, RN, Straznicky, NE, Sethi, P, Cohen, ND, Cerin, E, Lambert, GW, Owen, N, Kingwell, BA, Dunstan, DW. (2016) "Interrupting prolonged sitting with brief bouts of light walking or simple resistance activities reduces resting blood pressure and plasma noradrenaline in type 2 diabetes." Journal of Hypertension 34(12): 2376–82. doi.org/10.1097/HJH.0000000000001101

Fukushima, N, Kitabayashi, M, Kikuchi, H, Sasai, H, Oka, K, Nakata, Y, Tanaka, S, Inoue, S. (2018) "Comparison of accelerometer-measured sedentary behavior, and light- and moderate-to-vigorous-intensity physical activity in white- and blue-collar workers in a Japanese manufacturing plant." Journal of Occupational Health 60(3): 246–253. doi: 10.1539/joh.2017-0276-OA.

Helgadóttir, B, Forsell, Y, Hallgren, M, Möller, J, Ekblom, Ö. (2017) "Long-term effects of exercise at different intensity levels on depression: A randomized controlled trial." Prev Med 105: 37–46. doi: 10.1016/j.ypmed.2017.08.008.

Jackson, B, O'Connell, SE, Waheed, G, Munir, F. (2018) "Effectiveness of the stand more at (SMArT) work intervention: Cluster randomised controlled trial." BMJ 363: 3870. doi.org/10.1136/bmj.k3870

Kandola, A, Rees, J, Stubbs, B, Dunstan, DW, Genevieve GN, Hayes JF. (2020) "Breaking up excessive sitting with light activity." cms.wellcome.org/sites/default/files/2021-05/breaking-up-excessive-sitting-light-activity-wellcome-workplace-mental-health.pdf

Loh, R, Stamatakis, E, Folkerts, D, Allgrove, JE, Moir, HJ. (2020) "Effects of Interrupting Prolonged Sitting with Physical Activity Breaks on Blood Glucose, Insulin and Triacylglycerol Measures: A Systematic Review and Meta-analysis." Sports Medicine 50(20): 295–330. doi.org/10.1007/s40279-019-01183-w

Mackie, P, Weerasekara, I, Crowfoot, G, Janssen, H, Holliday, E, Dunstan, D, English, C. (2019) "What is the effect of interrupting prolonged sitting with frequent bouts of physical activity or standing on first or recurrent stroke risk factors? A scoping review." PLOS ONE 14(6): e0217981. doi.org/10.1371/journal.pone.0217981

Munir, F, Biddle, SJH, Davies, MJ, Dunstan, D, Esliger, D, Gray, LJ, Jackson, BR, O'Connell, SE, Yates, T, Edwardson, CL. (2018) "Stand More AT Work (SMArT Work): Using the behaviour change wheel to develop an intervention to reduce sitting time in the workplace." BMC Public Health 18, 319. doi.org/10.1186/s12889-018-5187-1

Prince, SA, Cardilli, L, Reed, JL, Saunders, TJ, Kite, C, Douillette, K, Fournier, K, Buckley, JPage (2020) "A comparison of self-reported and device measured sedentary behaviour in adults: A systematic review and meta-analysis." International Journal of Behavioral Nutrition and Physical Activity 17(1): 1–17. BioMed Central Ltd. doi.org/10.1186/s12966-020-00938-3

Straker, L, Abbott, RA, Heiden, M, Mathiassen, SEtoomingas, A. (2013) "Sit-stand desks in call centres: Associations of use and ergonomics awareness with sedentary behavior." Appl Ergon 44(4): 517–22. doi.org/10.1016/j.apergo.2012.11.001

Useful Resources

WEBSITES

www.pilatesatyourdesk.com

This is my website and home to my monthly subscription: "Move At Your Desk". All standing and seated movements are intended to be something you can slot into your working day. If you are looking for that extra prod then this monthly subscription includes lots of pre-recorded content, the option of a regular email reminding you to move, and several live 15-minute sessions per week for you to join. My website is also home to lots of articles and information that I have written over the years, as well as details of all of my online and in-person offerings (corporate workshops, 121 mat and equipment Pilates and group classes).

www.getbritainstanding.org

An initiative to get people moving more at work. You'll find lots of research and information about the benefits of sitting less all in one place.

www.drchatterjee.com

Home to "Feel Better Live More" podcast: a series of interviews with experts in the field of health and wellbeing.

www.balancedbody.com

For all things Pilates, equipment and accessories.

BOOKS

Self-Care for the Real World: Practical Self-Care Advice for Everyday Life by Nadia Narain and Katia Narain-Phillips

Tiny Habits: The Small Changes That Change Everything by BJ Fogg

Exercised by Daniel Lieberman

Return to Life Through Contrology by Joseph Pilates

GADGETS I USE

www.bellicon.com/gb_en
The home of the rebounder. This is what I bounce on at home!

uk.harmonidesk.com
The standing desk that I use and love because it the height can be adjusted.

CONTRIBUTORS

Emma Bray
www.emmabraypilates.co.uk

Sarah Woodhouse
www.sarahwoodhousepilates.com

Tessa Clist
www.arcpilates.com

Julie Driver
www.juliedriverpilates.com

Jenna Zaffino
www.jennazaffino.com

Grace Lillywhite
www.centredmums.com

Grace Hurry
www.gracehurry.com

Kath Pentecost
www.kathpentpilates.com

Fehmidah Munir

www.lboro.ac.uk/departments/ssehs/staff/fehmidah-munir/

Katharine Ayivor-Nygard

wearefullcircle.co

Carrie

www.instagram.com/carriespilares

Anya Hayes

www.instagram.com/mothers.wellness.toolkit

Index

A

abductors 103

ache between the shoulder
blades 147

aches and pains 145–9

active sitting 44–5

active standing 56–7

adductors 103

arm circles 159

arm lifting 70–1, 75

arm pulses 78–9

arms up and down 158

Ayivor-Nygard, Dr Katharine
33–5, 206

B

back flop 100, 191

belly breathing 143, 148

big and wide breaths 144, 148, 191

bones 18, 29–30

bone stacking 54

bottom pain 149

bottom shuffle 112–13

Bray, Emma 17, 184, 205

breathing 140–4

Bridge, Tannis 179

bum grippin 62, 104, 149

C

cactus arms 76, 147

cat/cow 98–9, 195

Charleston legs seated 120, 195

Chatterjee, Dr Rangan 32, 204

chest 69–82

Clist, Tessa 164–5, 205

COVID-19 9

D

dancing 169

door frame stretch 147, 162

Driver, Julie 52, 205

E

elbow circles 74, 192

elbows 72

elbows in, forearms out 159

elbow swimming 74, 146

extend the upper spine – lift collar
bones 97–8, 192

extension 89, 146, 147

F

Facegym 203
face massage 84
fascia 19, 20–2, 163
    Plantar fascia 19
feet 128–139, 166
Fletcher, Ron 7, 140
flexion 89, 90
flex your spine from bottom
    to top 96–7, 192
foot refresh 166
forward and back 132
front-of-neck stretch 86–7,
    148, 194

G

gluteus maximus 103
Goucher, Kara 184

H

hamstrings 103
hamstrings and inside thighs 113
hamstring stretches 117
    seated hamstring stretch, 117–18
    standing hamstring stretch 118–19
hands 136–9
Harmoni desk 51, 205

Hayes, Anya 170
head and neck alignment 85
head circles with eyes 85–6, 194
heel connection 53, 56–7
heel lifts 130–1, 134, 190
    both heels, 130
    single heel lifts, 130
    to your tip toes 131
herniated discs 88
hip hinge 114, 146
hip pain 149
hip stretch 122, 191, 193
hug a tree 77–8, 147
hug breaths 144
Hurry, Grace 49, 206
hypermobility 48
hyper-extension 72

I

infinity sign 139
inside outside 132
ironing board standing desk 163

J
jaw clenching 84
jazz hands 136
joints 18
    sacroiliac joint 43

K
Karate Kid meets Vogue 138
Kegel exercises 151
kitchen bench stretch 161
knee de-crankifier 167
kyphosis 89

L
lateral breathing 142, 146, 190, 194
leaning 55
leg crossing 43, 47
leg hanging 124–5, 149
legs 58–9, 102–127
lift and melt 73, 194
Lilywhite, Grace 150, 206
lower back pain 146
lower leg muscles 103
Loughborough University 24, 31

M
march 112, 195
Mexican wave 138

mighty yawn 80, 190, 194
morning routine 190
movement bank 28–9
Munir, Professor Fehmidah 24–5,
    31, 206
muscles 19, 29–30

N
neck 83–7
 neck and shoulder tension 194
neck pain 148
nervous system 19, 33–4
    vagus nerve 33–4
nodding 84

P
palm stretch 137
pelvic floor 150–151
pelvic pain 149
pelvic stability 108–9
pelvic tilts 105–6
pelvis 59, 88–9, 90, 102–127,
    150–153
Pentecost, Katherine 21, 206
Pez head 87
Pilates At Your Desk (PAYD) 7, 10,
    35, 38, 154, 172, 182–3, 186, 187,
    199, 203

Pilates for equestrians 52

Pilates, Joseph 7, 8, 88, 145, 204

plié with heel lifts 123

polishing the top of your halo
75–6, 147, 193

Plato 23

pregnancy 150–3

Q

quadriceps 103

R

rib breathing 146

robot 77

roll-down 126–127

roll your ankles 131

rotation 89, 93, 146, 147, 192

rotation with hands on knees
93–4, 190, 195

rotation with legs and arms in
a "V" 94–5, 192

routines for between meetings
191–2

S

sciatica 109–110, 149

seated lunge 116

seated squat 114–15, 191

self-massage 164–8

shake breaks 27–68, 146, 178,
191, 193

Shaw, George Bernard 177

shoulder circles 73–4, 193, 194

shoulder easer 168

shoulder circles 38, 147, 148, 195

shoulders 69–82

side-bending 89, 91, 92, 146,
147, 192

side-bend with arms over head, 92

single leg lift seated 119

sit bones 44–5, 106, 146, 149

skeleton 18

sofa back extension 162

spine 88–101

spondylolisthesis 88

spreading and lifting your toes
133–4

standing knee circles 121, 149, 191,
193

standing on one leg 120

Stand More AT (SMArT) Work
24–5, 31

star and ball 10, 101, 147, 190, 193

Stubbs, Dr Brendan 32

swimming 81–2

Swiss ball 51, 152–3

T

tennis balls 163–8

text neck 83–4

to the point 135

trampolines 170, 205

turning your head 86

typing 71

W

Williams, Sarah 107

wobble seat pad 51

Woodhouse, Sarah 37, 80, 205

World Health Organization 23, 26,
   30, 32–3

wrist rolls 137, 195

wrists 136–9

Z

Zaffino, Jenna 169, 205